Practical Doppler Ultrasound
for the
Clinician

Practical Doppler Ultrasound for the Clinician

Raymond L. Powis, Ph.D.
Quantum Medical Systems
Issaquah, Washington

and

Robert A. Schwartz, M.D.
Associate Professor of Surgery
State University of New York Health Science Center
Department of Surgery, Vascular Surgery Service
Syracuse, New York

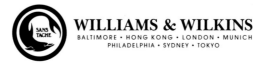

WILLIAMS & WILKINS
BALTIMORE · HONG KONG · LONDON · MUNICH
PHILADELPHIA · SYDNEY · TOKYO

Editors: Charles M. Mitchell and Timothy H. Grayson
Copy Editor: Starr Belsky
Production Coordinator: Kathleen C. Millet
Production and Design: Stony Run Publishing Services, Baltimore, Maryland
Cover Designer: Sheila Stoneham

Accurate indications, adverse reactions, and dosage schedules for drugs are provided in
this book, but it is possible that they may change. The reader is urged to review the package
information data of the manufacturers of the medications mentioned.

Printed in the United States of America

Library of Congress Cataloging in Publication Data

Powis, Raymond L.
    Practical Doppler ultrasound for the clinician / Raymond L. Powis and
Robert A. Schwartz.
      p.   cm.
    Includes bibliographical references and index.
    ISBN 0-683-06958-6
    1. Ultrasonics in medicine.   2. Doppler ultrasonography.   I. Schwartz,
Robert A., 1953–   .   II. Title
    [DNLM: 1. Ultrasonics. 2. Ultrasonography—instrumentation.
3. Ultrasonography—methods.   WB 289 P888p]
    RC857.U48P68   1991
    616.07'543—dc20
    DNLM/DLC
    for Library of Congress   91-7235
                                            CIP

91 92 93 94
1 2 3 4 5 6 7 8 9 10

This book is dedicated to our students
who showed that Doppler was not too far away to be known . . .

"Imagination is more important than knowledge."
—found in a fortune cookie

"But without knowledge, what is there to imagine?"
—the reader's retort

Preface

The title of this book is both specific and generic: specific in terms of "practical," and generic in terms of "clinician." Indeed, our clinician may be a physician, nurse, vascular technologist, echocardiographer, or sonographer, in short, anyone who places Doppler transducers on a patient and tries to read the results. And with each passing day, the number of Doppler users is growing, spreading into nearly every clinical niche in medicine.

The organization and presentation of information in this book emerged from an unusual crucible: short clinical workshops and seminars of one week or less. The test in these workshops is to portray information and connections for comprehension in two stages: a short-term functional grasp of the Doppler tool and its use, and a long-term insight into other applications and the interpretation of Doppler-dependent events. The first occurs in the workshop; the second occurs at home as the practitioner continues to use Doppler devices and thinks about results.

Within the growing range of Doppler ultrasound books now available, this one is neither an atlas of clinical presentations nor is it merely a detailed explanation of Doppler technology. Instead, the text centers on the connections between clinical applications and the technologies that make them possible. As a result, it is a good starting place for the new user of any Doppler device, including someone progressing from the simpler Doppler instruments to the more sophisticated duplex and color flow systems. Moreover, it is a profitable way to extend personal studies into the more advanced books on Doppler technology.

Because imagination plays such a central role in both understanding and using Doppler ultrasound, we have incorporated many figures to illustrate concepts and interactions. Indeed, errors and limitations in using Doppler devices often stem not from poor designs or from intractable patient conditions, but from the attitude and imagination of the user.

Although any chapter can be read on its own, the chapters are arrayed in a sequence to build logical connections among key ideas. They should be read in order on the first pass through the book.

Our shared fascination with Doppler ultrasound certainly comes from its vivid depiction of cardiovascular physiology in health and disease. Through this book, we invite others to join us in the ever changing, ever engaging world of Doppler ultrasound.

Raymond L. Powis, Ph.D.

Robert A. Schwartz, M.D.

Acknowledgments

Although we have not carried out a formal search for a Doppler gene, the evidence to date certainly suggests that none exists—especially in us. This book depended first of all on those who taught us, who shared information, coached, coaxed, and chided until we were on the right course. How can we name them all? We cannot, but that makes them no less contributors. We extend a special thanks to them all.

On a more direct level, we did get some unstinting support when we needed more than what was at hand. Quantum Medical Systems, Issaquah, Washington, Advanced Technology Labs, Bothell, Washington, and the University of Washington Department of Surgery quickly and generously responded to requests for help. We also thank Katey Millet and Starr Belsky for managing and editing the book into final form. And, of course, we would like to thank Williams & Wilkins for their patience and encouragement when progress seemed to slow to a crawl.

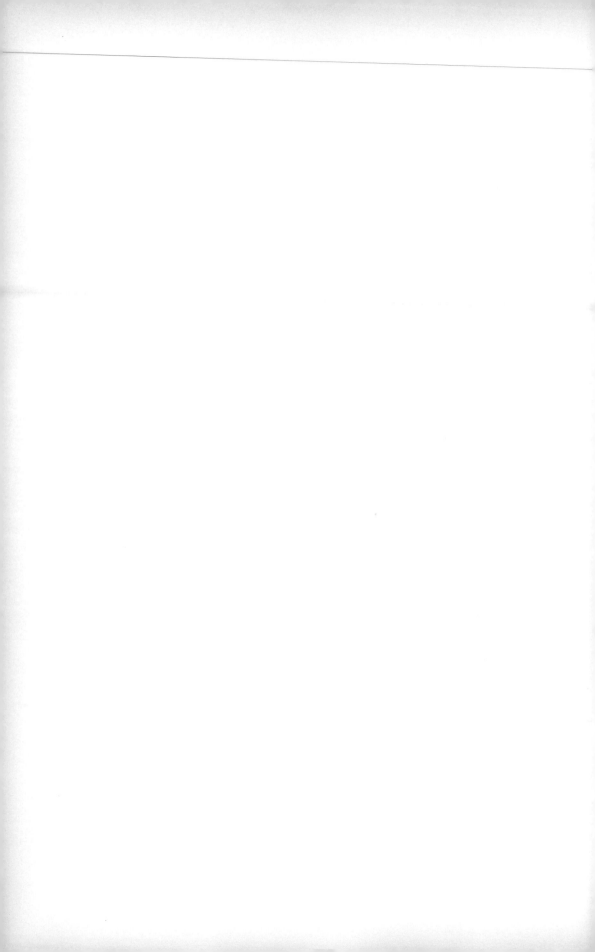

Contents

Preface / vii
Acknowledgments / ix

1   Gaining a Clinical Perspective / 1

2   In Search of a Global View / 9

3   The Tissue–Ultrasound Interaction / 17

4   Building a Model of Blood Flow / 35

5   The Doppler Equation as a Tool / 63

6   Primary Steps in Doppler Signal Processing / 75

7   Signal-Processing Details / 89

8   Duplex Imaging and Other Advanced Techniques / 109

9   Linking Doppler Displays with Physical Events / 133

10   Quantitation and Doppler Ultrasound / 155

Index / 179

1

Gaining a
Clinical Perspective

You may have either reviewed the table of contents or already leafed through this text and noticed the equations and line drawings reminiscent of a physics textbook. You may feel certain that this esoterica could not possibly relate to clinical medicine. We hope to challenge that skepticism and persuade you to read the other nine chapters, and we hope this chapter will offer you, as a clinician, some justification for your efforts.

Doppler ultrasound technology is now an integral part of clinical medicine in almost every subspecialty. Systems extend from the simple continuous wave Doppler device, used in conjunction with an inflatable cuff to measure blood pressure, to the sophisticated color flow equipment used in echocardiography and vascular imaging. The impact of this technology is irrefutable. To the majority of clinicians using Doppler ultrasound, these space-age machines are nothing more than magical black boxes that spew out reproducible pieces of numerical clinical wisdom. In truth, these devices interact with the human organism, process the product of that interaction, and then produce data that are clinically valuable. In every step of the process, interpretive error awaits the unwary and can lead to a poor patient outcome. In other words, if the clinician misuses the technology or misunderstands its output, it is usually the patient who suffers. This is the way of clinical medicine. Some practical examples can illustrate our meaning.

Use and Misuse of the Hand-Held Doppler Device

One of the most common uses of Doppler ultrasound is to determine the presence or absence of blood flow. The tool is a small, 5- to 8-MHz continuous wave (CW) Doppler ultrasound device, available at almost every nursing station throughout an average hospital. These Doppler devices are often used in conjunction with a standard blood pressure cuff to measure systolic blood pressure. When the cuff pressure falls below the systolic arterial blood pressure, the CW Doppler device detects the arterial blood flow passing beyond the cuff. This technique is second nature to most nurses and physicians who care for pediatric patients or critically ill patients in shock. In these patients, hearing Korotkoff sounds with a conventional stethoscope is difficult or even impossible. Could such a simple technique be prone to error? To answer that question, let's look at the two essential steps in the technique.

Initially, the transducer emits ultrasound into the tissue and echoes return to the apparatus for processing. The first error that often occurs at this early step is failure to make a good acoustical coupling. All ultrasound Doppler devices transmit sound energy into the body and receive echoes from the aggregates of red blood cells. Getting the acoustic energy into and out of the body requires a coupling material between the plastic membrane that covers the ultrasound transducer and the tissues.

Unfortunately, the Doppler user often applies either an inadequate amount of acoustical gel or a gel made for other purposes such as making electrocardiograms. Some of the more innovative substitutions include lubricant jelly, electrical conduction gel, or even occasionally anesthetic gel. In fact, such compromises in acoustic coupling can make the detection of blood flow impossible. If the user is lucky enough to detect flow, the results will often underestimate the systolic blood pressure because the true initial blood movements are lost. These small echo signals simply never make it through the poor coupling into the Doppler device for processing. This error is easy to see when the patient happens to have an invasive monitor such as an arterial pressure line to provide more direct values.

A second sort of error occurs when the user misunderstands how the Doppler device processes returning echo signals for frequency shift information. Chapter 6 explains how CW Doppler devices compare the frequency of the transmitted ultrasound waves to the reflected or returning ultrasound waves. From this comparison, the frequency shift caused by the moving blood becomes the audio signal so familiar to most clinicians.

A fundamental Doppler principle, however, is the need for an angle of less than 90° between the ultrasound beam and the moving blood. In other words, the beam cannot be perpendicular to the moving blood. If the examiner happens to hold the transducer perpendicular to the vessel, then no useful Doppler shift frequencies will appear in the audio output.

In the clinical setting, this error occurs when an examiner unthinkingly moves the angle of insonation close to 90° in a hypotensive patient. The combination of a steep Doppler angle and low blood velocities may give no audible Doppler shift, yet simply setting the angle to 45° can restore the Doppler sounds. Indeed, merely tilting the transducer can change a patient's appearance from a hypotensive individual requiring pharmacological manipulation to a normotensive individual. In this instance, simply understanding how the ultrasound is emitted, propagated, processed, and received can eliminate several clinical errors.

Another sort of error can come from a physician who misinterprets adequately transmitted and received ultrasound information. For example, the CW Doppler is often used by the physician not only to detect the presence and absence of flow, but also to assess its velocity. Patients with peripheral arterial occlusive disease such as atherosclerosis are popular targets for this technique. These atherosclerotic patients frequently do not have palpable peripheral pulses. As a result, a hand-held CW Doppler device can be quite helpful in assessing the severity of any flow disorder.

A very common mistake in this evaluation is to associate the volume of the audio output with volumetric flow. For example, one often hears the novice observe that the patient has excellent blood flow to an extremity based on a loud pulsatile audio output. In truth, the audio output loudness is unrelated to the volumetric flow in an artery. The audio output volume is identical to sound amplification in a radio. Clearly, turning up the volume control of a radio does not change the notes of music. Indeed, loud Doppler sounds are merely sounds undergoing significant amplification. As other parts of this text show, frequency shifts correlate directly with flow velocity. A patient may have loud, high-pitched Doppler flow signals due to intense vasospasm or areas of arterial stenosis where the volumetric flow may be quite low. Such a misinterpretation of Doppler information could lead a clinician away from identifying or acting appropriately when an organ or a limb might be in jeopardy. The CW Doppler is a blind device, unable to ascertain the size of the vessel in its beam, and cannot tell the clinician about the adequacy of flow needed to keep an extremity alive. Let's take a closer look at the aptness of these thoughts in the context of a familiar clinical setting.

Physicians frequently face patients who have recently suffered a profound myocardial infarction. Along with the infarction, these patients often have systemic atherosclerosis and subsequently chronic stenoses or occlusions in the major arteries of their extremities. Because these obstructions are chronic, the patients routinely develop sufficient collateral circulation to keep their extremities alive. Patients with a recent myocardial infarction are typically in cardiogenic shock, raising a clinical dilemma: what is the etiology of an ischemic extremity? Complicating the decision is the fact that myocardial infarctions can generate peripheral embolization from blood clots and thrombi that originate along the noncontractile myocardium in a ventricle. These emboli end up in the peripheral arterial tree, acutely occluding peripheral arteries and threatening a limb with acute injury because of hypoperfusion. This situation requires therapeutic intervention.

In contrast, the same hypotensive patient, in cardiogenic shock, may have ischemic appearing extremities from chronic occlusions and low cardiac output. The limb appears ischemic because the collateral vascular beds have a higher vascular resistance than the original arterial tree, which is now stenotic or occluded.

The character of the Doppler sounds from a CW device would be distinctly different for these two clinical situations. Embolic obstruction causes low-velocity signals in the distal extremity, whereas cardiogenic shock with vasospasm causes high-velocity or high-resistance signals. Along with the Doppler sounds, the therapeutic intervention is significantly different for these two different disease states. The Doppler sound patterns are predictive in most circumstances for the underlying pathology. The accuracy, though, and the diagnostic value of the Doppler devices rides completely on an understanding of the technology and its interaction with the human organism expressing the pathophysiology of vascular disease.

Doppler Ultrasound Technology Is Changing the Practice of Medicine

Doppler ultrasound technology is continuing to spread within the hospital environment. Most of the clinical disciplines use Doppler analysis of some sort in routine clinical practice. In addition, Doppler information is even an integral part of the diagnostic algorithm that justifies invasive procedures and therapy. The attraction is clear. This diagnostic modality offers minimal patient risk for procedures that have an excellent, accurate diagnostic capability.

Cardiology is a good place to look at some of these clinical changes. In the era prior to echocardiography, cardiologists were forced to consider every patient with a cardiac murmur as a candidate for diagnostic cardiac catheterization with its significant morbidity. Echocardiography changed that. The majority of patients with cardiac murmurs have the source of those murmurs correctly diagnosed with ultrasound. Now, patients not requiring therapeutic intervention seldom undergo the relatively dangerous diagnostic testing of invasive cardiac catheterization.

Beyond the screening value of echocardiography, clinicians are now able to quantify several aspects of cardiac disease. As Chapter 10 illustrates, a modified Bernoulli equation has become a way to quantify the degree of valvular stenosis and the remaining valve area for stenotic cardiac valves. Routinely, patients with aortic valve stenosis are followed using these calculations until symptoms and Doppler findings suggest that intervention is warranted. Doppler-derived estimations of cardiac output provide a very real clinical utility.

The vascular clinician has followed an almost parallel course for handling patients with carotid occlusive disease. Well before an angiogram is necessary, a noninvasive examination of the cervical cerebrovasculature is carried out with a combination of B-mode imaging and Doppler ultrasound (duplex imaging). Now, patients who are free of cervical atherosclerosis rarely undergo angiography. Before Strandness and coworkers[1] established the clinical accuracy of this application of ultrasound, many patients with normal vessels underwent angiography with its significant morbidity and mortality. This morbidity included the devastating complication of stroke in patients free of atherosclerosis in their cerebrovasculature. Clearly, correct use of this new tool eliminates the diagnostic need to perform invasive testing without just cause.

Sophisticated Equipment Produces Sophisticated Artifacts

As Doppler ultrasound devices continue to improve, producing better depictions of anatomy and blood flow, investigators continue to expand the use of the technology into more challenging clinical problems.[2–8] These new, clearer images, however, can give a false sense of security about their clinical accuracy. A high-quality image does not prevent errors predicated on an inadequate understanding of the interface between a patient and the interrogating technology.

A fertile area for misinterpretation of Doppler ultrasound data is in carotid artery duplex imaging. A small but not insignificant portion of the patient population has quite tortuous or anomalous carotid arteries. These anatomical variations can lead to a misdiagnosis of stenosis in an otherwise normal (but tortuous) artery. Scanning these patients produces confusing images of arterial parts because of the vessel's tortuosity. Vessel segments that are nearly perpendicular to the incident ultrasound clearly appear in the B-mode image. Segments that are parallel, or nearly so, to the transmitted ultrasound are often lost in a fog of gray-scale noise. These vessel segments (which may be the whole distal internal carotid artery) vanish because they present no reflective surface to the ultrasound beam. Without a vessel wall in view, the sonographer cannot accurately position the Doppler beam using the B-mode image. The practical alternative is to sample blindly using a wide-range gate in the area just distal to the visualized artery. Because the flow in this portion of the artery is close to parallel to the ultrasound beam, it effectively has a 0° angle of insonation. Despite the normal flow velocities in the artery, all of the Doppler frequency components are elevated because of the acute scanning angle.

Along with the high frequencies, the tortuous carotid artery also leads to non-parabolic flow patterns that create a wide range of velocities and consequently spectral broadening. This combination of spectral broadening and high Doppler frequencies is the primary criterion for stenosis in patients with atherosclerotic carotid occlusive disease. Differentiating a stenosis from a tortuous, unnarrowed artery requires knowing the angle of insonation. The criteria for determining percent stenosis using Doppler-derived flow events are based on a known angle of insonation. And, of course, blind Doppler sampling offers no known angle of insonation. Understanding the rules of gathering Doppler flow information along with normal anatomical variance and the pathophysiology of atherosclerotic occlusive disease can prevent confusion or a wrong conclusion.

Just as an unsuspected acute angle can cause problems, so can relatively large angles of insonation. To help create some uniformity in interpreting carotid duplex ultrasonography, physicians have moved from frequency- to velocity-specific criteria. Velocity-specific criteria used to estimate percent stenosis should remain uniform, whether the information comes from a 5- , 7.5- , or even 10-MHz transmission frequency.

Although standardization to velocity criteria removes some confusion due to the different transmitted frequencies, it raises another set of problems for the uninitiated Doppler user. The need to set the correct angle of insonation has not gone away. It is not uncommon for the angle assignment to vary as much as $\pm$ 5° from the true angle, even in linear-appearing arteries. This occurs not because of a poor operator angle setup, but because of nonaxial flow within the arteries as they branch and turn. At 72°, a 3° error leads to a 15% to 20% error in the velocity calculation. But a 3° error when the angle is close to 85° creates a greater than 100% error in the velocity calculation. Large discrepancies can occur between a Doppler-derived percent stenosis and angiographic data simply because of these steep Doppler angles.

Atherosclerotic plaque can be both highly echogenic and attenuating from calcification and the fibrous components of the plaque. As the dense plaque components become more reflective, they create echoes several thousand times larger than the echoes from the moving red blood cells. Often a sonographer will try to obtain flow data in the lumen of a highly echogenic atherosclerotic vessel. Although the amplitude of reflected ultrasound is sufficient to delineate the vessel walls, the plaque and vessel attenuate the low-amplitude reflected signals utilized for Doppler flow detection. Without the Doppler flow signals, these vessels appear to be occluded, based on the absence of detectable flow. In reality, the highly echogenic and attenuating plaque materials have reduced the already weaker signals from the flowing blood. Understanding that the echo amplitudes processed for Doppler are significantly smaller than the amplitudes from reflected ultrasound for the B-mode image can prevent confusing no flow signals with no flow.

Color Doppler Ultrasound Imaging—The Next Step

The increasing capabilities and sophistication of computer technology have not only changed the personal computer, they have changed ultrasound. It is now possible to represent not only the amplitudes of signals from the tissues, but also the flow events from the same sampling sites of an ultrasound image. The result is equipment that will simultaneously create a B-mode image of anatomy and a Doppler ultrasound image of the flow characteristics throughout the scanning field. Flow appears as color, with a specific color representing flow direction and a change in hue or saturation representing Doppler shift frequencies within the flow.

Although the images appear familiar to the clinician and somewhat reminiscent of his Grant's *Atlas of Anatomy* textbook,[9] this form of processing actually increases the complexity of interpretation. At the same time, the expanded complexity of the image also increases the number of possible artifacts and the possibility of making a clinically relevant error. This can be illustrated with a simple example.

Detecting the presence or absence of blood flow should be a relatively simple and uniformly accurate activity with a color Doppler system. That is certainly true in the majority of but not all clinical situations.

One unfortunate complication that occurs with transarterial catheterization is the development of a pseudoaneurysm at the puncture wound in the artery. The pulsatile arterial pressure keeps the wound open, driving blood out into the false cavity adjacent to the artery. During diastole, the elastic components of the adjacent tissue drive the extraluminal blood back into the vessel. The pseudoaneurysm either gradually expands, requiring surgical repair, or spontaneously clots, forming a hematoma.

Prior to duplex ultrasonography, the clinician was forced to utilize another transarterial invasive procedure, arteriography, to diagnose the presence or absence of a periarterial pseudoaneurysm. From the patient's perspective, it was often difficult to tolerate a second procedure that was reminiscent of the original cause of the current problem.

Duplex ultrasonography could detect extraluminal flow with a characteristic spectral signal. Color Doppler imaging, on the other hand, provides more anatomical detail, including the presence of extraluminal flow, site of the arterial puncture, and anatomy of the native arteries, all without angiography.[10] Clinical correlations between the image and pseudoaneurysms at the time of surgical repair showed the technique to be quite reliable. Moreover, long-term follow-up of pseudoaneurysms that had appeared to resolve and of periarterial hematomas without extraluminal blood flow demonstrated the precision of the technique. Color Doppler imaging appeared to be an ideal tool to discriminate between the pseudoaneurysm and the periarterial hematoma with sufficient information to avoid angiography. Within all this success, however, lay the foundation for an error.

Following an intra-arterial injection of illegal pharmaceuticals, a patient presented with a tender, pulsatile, periarterial mass. The color Doppler image showed Doppler signals adjacent to the underlying artery. Here was a discrete mass with color pixels adjacent to the artery. Clearly, it was a pseudoaneurysm. At surgery, the patient had periarterial abscess with no evidence of pseudoaneurysm formation or extraluminal blood flow. How could this error have happened?

This error hinged on a misunderstanding of how the color Doppler image is formed. The proteinaceous material within the abscess produced sufficiently strong echoes to be detected. Secondly, the pulsation of the artery adjacent to the abscess transmitted motion to the fluid within the mass. Thus, the echo signals had both strength and motion, with sufficient movement to generate a frequency shift and thus detectable Doppler information.

In retrospect, the abscess did not have the hemodynamic characteristics of a pseudoaneurysm, with inflow and outflow of blood. The images of the abscess merely showed the waves of energy being transmitted through the fluid rather than a characteristic hydrodynamic pattern. Knowing about the hemodynamics of human disease states, the tissue-ultrasound interaction, and ultrasound signal processing are essential to avoid such errors.

Summary and Digressions

Ultrasound imaging equipment has permeated almost every clinical discipline in medicine. Anesthesiologists monitor CW Doppler signals aimed at the heart, seeking sounds reminiscent of air entrapment in an upright anesthetized patient undergoing a neurosurgical procedure. At the other end of the body, the urologist is utilizing Doppler ultrasound to determine the source of impotence.[11]

Duplex ultrasonography and now color Doppler ultrasound imaging are reliable modalities for depicting atherosclerotic cervical cerebrovascular disease. Few patients go to angiography without ultrasound screening. The rationale for this algorithm is that a reliable screening test can separate all the normal individuals from candidates for more dangerous investigative methods, as well as remove those individuals who would least benefit from invasive procedures. This practice is logical if the screening test is reasonably accurate.

Duplex ultrasonography of the carotid arteries has been shown to be sufficiently accurate to fill this role as a screening test, with sensitivities and selectivities greater than 90% in experienced hands.[12] This level of accuracy rests on the assumption that the individual interpreting the Doppler ultrasound data is aware of the relationship between ultrasound physics and clinical medicine.

This insertion of ultrasound as an intermediate step to more dangerous procedures is apparent in other disciplines. Few patients go for cardiac catheterization to evaluate valvular heart disease without duplex echocardiography. Moreover, in the vascular department, color Doppler imaging is quickly replacing intravenous contrast venography for the diagnosis of deep venous thrombosis.

The clinical applications of ultrasound continue to grow. Soon, nearly every clinician will use the output from ultrasound technology to manage patients. Even if the clinician does not apply the technology personally, the need to be able to interpret the results of the data remains. Artifacts and interpretation must be part of every physician's knowledge base. Inaccurate diagnosis based on inappropriate interpretation of ultrasound data can lead to devastating consequences. The physics and engineering necessary for understanding ultrasound technology are foreign to most physicians, but they are not impossible to learn and use. We are certain that any efforts to understand the tool and its interaction with your patients will be rewarded with improved diagnostic capabilities as well as a lower incidence of diagnostic artifacts.

References

1. Blackshear, WM, Phillips, DJ, Thiele, BL, Hirsch, JH, Chikos, PM, Strandness, DE. Detection of carotid occlusive disease by ultrasonic imaging and pulsed Doppler spectrum analysis. *Surgery* 86:698–706, 1979.
2. Schwartz, RA, Peterson, GJ, Noland, KA, et al. Intraoperative duplex scanning following carotid artery reconstruction: A valuable tool. *J Vasc Surg* 7:620–624, 1988.
3. Langsfeld, M, Nepute, J, Hershey, FB, et al. The use of deep duplex scanning to predict hemodynamically significant aortoiliac stenoses. *J Vasc Surg* 7:395–399, 1988.
4. Igidbashian, VN, Mitchell, DG, Middleton, WD, et al. Iatrogenic femoral arteriovenous fistula: Diagnosis with color Doppler imaging. *Radiology* 170:749–752, 1989.
5. Mitchell, DG, Needleman, JE, Bezzi, M, et al. Femoral artery pseudoaneurysm: Diagnosis with conventional ultrasound and color Doppler ultrasound. *Radiology* 165:687–690, 1987.

6. Kohler, TR, Zierler, RE, Martin, RL, et al. Noninvasive diagnosis of renal artery stenosis by duplex scanning. *J Vasc Surg* 4:450–456, 1986.

7. Jager, K, Bollinger, A, Valli, C, and Ammann, R. Measurement of mesenteric blood flow by duplex scanning. *J Vasc Surg* 3:462–469, 1986.

8. Comerato, AJ, Katz, ML, Greenwald, LL, et al. Venous duplex imaging: Should it replace hemodynamic tests for deep venous thrombosis. *J Vasc Surg* 11:53–59, 1990.

9. Grant, JCB. *An Atlas of Anatomy,* ed 9. Baltimore: Williams & Wilkins, 1991.

10. Schwartz, RA, Kerns, DB, Mitchell, DG. Color Doppler ultrasound imaging in iatrogenic arterial injuries. *Am J Surg* (in press).

11. Shabsingh, R, Fishman, IJ, Quesada, ET, et al. Evaluation of vasculogenic erectile impotence using penile duplex ultrasonography. *J Urol* 142:1469–1474, 1989.

12. Zwiebel, WJ, Austin, CW, Sackett, JF, et al. Correlation of high resolution, B-mode and continuous wave Doppler sonography with arteriography in the diagnosis of carotid stenosis. *Radiology* 149:523–532, 1983.

2

In Search of a Global View

So often, our understanding of an object or process is governed more by our emotional reaction to the words used to describe it than by any real complexity in the object or process itself. This is clearly the case for Doppler ultrasound. Our reaction to the words "Doppler physics" seems to swamp any attempts at explanation. The Doppler effect, its special signal processing, methods in drawing diagnostic conclusions from Doppler information, or just setting up a Doppler sonograph are all just too difficult. Indeed, "Doppler physics" is a special incantation that turns an eager audience of students into lightly sedated, glassy-eyed humans, convinced they are unable to learn such a difficult topic.

This response, though frustrating, is understandable and comes from two sources. First, formal courses in physics have been the centers for "aversion therapy" in our educational system, designed to make sure everyone hates physics. Second, most of the information printed about Doppler ultrasound looks like an engineering or physics Ph.D. thesis. Given these conditions, how could Doppler ultrasound ever become a success in the medical community? Despite these impediments, it has become the most rapidly growing application of diagnostic ultrasound today.

Impediments aside, the reasons for this steady growth of Doppler ultrasound are all quite clear. Doppler provides information about body physiology and pathology that is otherwise hard to obtain. And in spite of its reputation for being difficult to learn and use, the diagnostic value of Doppler continues steadily to draw new users. But some relief to the problem is at hand. We show in this book that Doppler science may be different from the way we normally think about the world, but it is not too difficult to master and use. And it is the contrast between the two words "different" and "difficult" that fuels our approach here. The goal, in the end, is to develop a thoughtful, different approach to understanding and using Doppler ultrasound. And getting there requires a global view of some of the events and ideas.

As a global view unfolds in this chapter, a newcomer to Doppler ultrasound will find many words and concepts that are new. They will fall into place later in the book with definitions and examples. And after reading the remainder of the book, it might be instructive to read this chapter again.

Viewing Reality

Psychologists tell us that we think with an internal, mental model of the outside world. This model produces a set of expectations for us about how the world works. Confusion reigns when events fall outside these expectations or when we have no expectations to evaluate events we may be witnessing.

This is certainly true in diagnostic ultrasound. Imaging the body's interior requires a three-dimensional mental model of the organ boundaries and the internal organization of each structure. Deviations from expected images usually generate a series of small experiments to determine the size, shape, position, texture, and dynamics of any anomalies as well as of the organs themselves. Such a model can do the same thing for Doppler ultrasound.

As we move through the various parts of Doppler ultrasound, each of these parts will be used to form an effective mental model of events. From the model will come expectations about such things as scanning techniques and the Doppler signal results, how logically to set up a Doppler sonograph, and strategies in using one of the most effective tools in Doppler ultrasound: the Doppler equation. Like the imaging goals of size, shape, position, texture, and dynamics, a set of Doppler goals will evolve that will help us look at and think about the Doppler ultrasound outputs.

The Doppler Effect in General

One of the first impediments to thinking about Doppler ultrasound is that it deals with things in motion. When most of us visualize something in our minds, it is a static picture. The Doppler effect, however, depends upon motion and patterns of motion, and this is an unfamiliar way of thinking about things.

In simple terms, the Doppler effect is the apparent change in pitch of a wave when relative motion exists between a moving wave-source and an observer. When no relative motion exists, no change in wave frequency occurs. As relative motion increases, however, the changes in wave frequency also increase. Thus, changes in frequency and the amount of change are linked directly to this relative motion. It is the value of the closing velocity, that is, how rapidly the source and observer are closing on one another, that explicitly produces the frequency change. Importantly, the motion information is hidden not in the wave frequency itself, but in the *change* in frequency. This change in frequency is called the Doppler shift frequency. The exact nature of this direct link can be found in the Doppler equation, which is the center of a more detailed discussion later.

The Doppler effect in ultrasound sets up an unexpectedly useful relationship. The primary target for the ultrasonic inquiry is the red blood cell, which moves through the various vascular compartments, passively following the local hydrodynamics. The typical ultrasonic frequencies and blood velocities within the body's vascular compartments combine to form Doppler shifts that fall within the human audio spectrum. And that condition sets up the first form of Doppler signal analysis: listening to the Doppler signals. Clearly, listening to the Doppler signals can place an observer in intimate contact with vascular events. Still, the representation of these events is coded into an unfamiliar audio signal.

The tool, however, can begin to shape our thinking. As we look at individual vascular compartments with Doppler devices, it is easy to think of the vascular system as a series of isolated tubes. In truth, the cardiovascular system is a large, complicated, extended organ. The tissue within this organ may be fluid, but considering its physical, functional, and biochemical character, blood carries all the traits of a true tissue. Furthermore, nerves, hormones, and local tissue level chemicals all produce controls for the system. The vascular system changes its tissue (blood) distribution based on need and carries out local reactions to injury and disease.

Supplying energy for most of the system's mechanically based activities is the heart. It is an artificial division to look at the vascular system and forget the heart as the source of hydrodynamic energy, or look at the heart and forget the vascular system into which it pumps. Aiding this egalitarian view of the cardiovascular system is the simple fact that the events producing the Doppler shift signal are the same for both the heart and the blood vessels. And in the end, viewing the cardiovascular system as an extended organ will give greater meaning to the events depicted in the Doppler signal output.

The Doppler Effect in Nature

Because "Doppler" is a man's name (Christian Johann Doppler, 1803–1853), it is easy to believe that humans invented the Doppler effect for their own purposes. Like so many other natural effects exploited by other living things within an adaptive biological community, the Doppler effect is widely used within the animal world. One successful user is, of course, the bat, which has almost become the official symbol of ultrasound in general.

Looking at the biological use of the Doppler effect brings us to the well-studied Panamanian mustache bat.[1] This particular bat locates and characterizes flying insects and calculates an interception course using the insect's range, its direction of flight, and its relative speed of flight. The speed calculation uses the Doppler effect.

Like many of our current duplex ultrasound systems, the bat does not carry out a Doppler-dependent calculation and a range determination at the same time.[2] This mutual exclusion of Doppler processing and echo ranging illustrates a similar problem in diagnostic ultrasound: the requirements for obtaining Doppler and echo-ranging information are different. These differences can be traced to the form of the transmitted ultrasound and the internal echo-signal processing. Thus, as we do, the bat uses two different forms of pulses for Doppler processing and echo ranging.

The Panamanian mustache bat uses ultrasound in the 50 to 65 kHz range for both echo ranging and Doppler.[1] These frequencies produce wave lengths in air of 6.6 to 5.0 mm, at a propagation velocity of 330 m/s. The bat transmits a series of monotonic bursts and examines the changes in echo frequency to determine the velocity of the target.[2] The bat then uses a series of bursts that chirp in frequency.[2] Changes in the character of the echo signal as a function of frequency give the bat information about the characteristics of the insect target. In this manner, the bat not only determines range, direction, and velocity, but also some of the physical characteristics of the target.

The length of the ultrasonic burst used by the mustache bat is about 1,000 times longer than those used in diagnostic ultrasound. For example, a monotonic burst for determining velocity can be from 5,000 to 30,000 μs long.[1] In comparison, diagnostic, pulsed Doppler ultrasound uses pulses only 1 to 2 μs long. Although a long burst length blurs the spatial resolving qualities of echo ranging, it does provide two benefits: first, it increases the amount of returning energy from a physically small target, improving the signal-to-noise ratio; and second, the length of the burst determines the lowest Doppler shift frequency. The lowest Doppler shift frequency, in turn, sets the lowest velocity resolvable by the Doppler system. In general, blood moves at higher velocities than flying insects, and the bat's longer sonic bursts better accommodate these lower flying velocities.

A question essential to the Doppler signal processing is how the bat determines the Doppler shift frequencies in the returning echoes. Accurate determination of small shifts in frequency would require some very sharp, neuronal frequency filters within the bat's central nervous system. Rather than reading the return frequency for its frequency shift, however, the bat uses a better controlled and easier reading mechanism. The bat's central nervous system is set to its central transmitting frequency, typically 65 kHz.[3] A returning echo with a different frequency prompts a new frequency for the transmit signal to restore the echo signal to 65 kHz.[3] Thus, an echo shifted up in frequency prompts a downward shift in the next transmit burst; an echo shifted down in frequency prompts an upward shift in the next transmit burst. The amount of frequency correction measures the Doppler shift frequency, and with it, how the target is moving in space.

After the monotonic bursts, the mustache bat emits a series of chirps that last 2,000 to 3,000 μs.[2] The chirps begin at 65 kHz and decrease to 55 kHz. Just how the bat carries out the analysis of the chirped signals is not yet entirely clear. Analysis of scattering signals shows that they can change amplitude in proportion to the frequency squared, cubed, or even to the fourth power. However the bats perform this analysis, the chirp provides not only an accurate determination of range and direction, but also rather detailed information about the nature of the target (insect). Bats trained in captivity, for example, can learn to discriminate between very similar yet subtly different targets.[4]

Despite the long wavelengths and extended bursts, the bat has an effective resolution of about 1 mm in air[4] and seems able to characterize a target with greater clarity than diagnostic ultrasound, which typically has a resolution of 1.5 to 3.0 mm. And currently we have a very limited ability to characterize tissue.

The phrase "seeing with sound" has acquired greater meaning in light of examinations of the bat's central nervous system: studies show that the audio portion mimics the visual cortex of other mammals.[3] This sort of rigid, high-level organization suggests that bats may form a three-dimensional acoustic image of the target in their brain. This image could include many of the discriminative capabilities attributed to vision. A comparison of bat and diagnostic ultrasound capabilities and parameters appears in Table 2–1.

Table 2–1.   Bat and Diagnostic Ultrasound Capabilities and Parameters

	Diagnostic ultrasound	Mustache bat
Frequencies	2–10 MHz	50–65 KHz
Transmission medium	Biological tissue	Air
Propagation velocity	1540 m/s	330 m/s
Medium attenuation	0.9 dB/cm/MHz (avg)	12 dB/cm/(MHz)^2
Wavelength	0.77–0.15 mm	6.6–5.0 mm
Burst length	1–6 μs	5,000–30,000 μs
Object size resolution	1 mm	1 mm

Doppler Application Goals: Source, Form, Frequency, and Direction

Through years of experience, the ultrasound community has developed a specific set of imaging goals: to determine the size, shape, position, texture, and dynamics of organs and structures within the body. These goals are more than a series of end points for the scans. They define a way of thinking about the scanning process itself and determine what the image must include to be of diagnostic value. These goals even influence the internal design of the imaging sonograph.[5]

A similar set of goals exist for Doppler ultrasound. Like the goals in ultrasonic imaging, they are more than just a group of end points for the Doppler scanning process: they provide a method of processing the Doppler output for clinical conclusions and affect the basic signal processing design within the Doppler sonograph. These logical goals are to determine the source of the Doppler signals; the form of these signals over time and space; the frequency content of the signals over time; and the direction of flow over time (Table 2–2). We consider them briefly here, but in more detail later in the book as the discussion links the various elements of Doppler ultrasound together.

Source

A central problem in using Doppler ultrasound in the cardiovascular system is that the latter is a large, complex, extended organ. In response to the needs of various organs, vessels feeding major vascular beds often have flow characteristics that are quite different. The simplest example is the markedly different flow through an artery and a vein. Clearly, flow through the heart differs from flow through small peripheral vessels, and the internal and external carotid arteries have very different flow cycles. Disease, however, can change flow to such an extent that its characteristics alone will not facilitate discrimination among different vessels. Therefore, both external and internal landmarks are needed to define the vessel producing the Doppler signals.

In general, knowing the source of the Doppler signals sets out the expected flow patterns. When these patterns change, disease may be present somewhere within a vessel. Changes can also indicate whether the system has compensated for disease by increasing flow through existing channels or by elaborating new collateral channels. Thus, knowing the source of the Doppler signals and what to expect under normal circumstances makes indications of disease and physiological compensation readily apparent.

This need to know the echo-signal source is so central to drawing conclusions about the cardiovascular system that it has shaped the basic design of the sonograph, its fundamental signal processing, and its elaboration into increasingly complex systems. Even simple continuous wave Doppler transducers have been physically modified to

Table 2–2.   Imaging Goals and Doppler Goals

Imaging goals	Doppler goals
Size	Source
Shape	Form
Position	Frequency
Texture	Direction
Dynamics	

determine the source of the Doppler signals. Pulsed Doppler systems have included M-mode and real-time B-mode imaging to determine the source of the signals. Indeed, the very reason for designing a pulsed Doppler was to determine uniquely the sources of the Doppler shift signals. When unusual results appear, the first clinical question is still: where did these Doppler signals come from?

Form

The energy that moves the blood through a vascular compartment is pulsatile. The physical shape of the flow response to this energy provides some direct evidence about physiological and pathological events within a vascular compartment. The shape of the flow velocities over time is determined not only by the presence of disease, but also by the physical characteristics of the vascular channels themselves.[6]

Form includes more than just the shape of events that divide the heart cycle into systole and diastole. Additional parameters include the rise time, maximum value, and changes in amplitude. A number of pulsatility measures give information about conditions within a vessel feeding a vascular bed as well as conditions within the bed itself. Two traditional examples of these indices are the so-called pulsatility index and Pourcelot's ratio.[7,8]

The form of the flow over time, however, is only part of the useful information. Other techniques that show in detail the patterns of flow through a compartment provide a spatial characterization of flow.[9,10] Thus, to be complete, the form of the flow must include not only temporal, but also spatial characteristics.

Frequency

The frequency components of a Doppler shift signal contain information on how the contributors to flow are changing over time. First, the spread of frequencies expresses the range of velocities passing through the sample volume. Second, the amplitude of a frequency component is proportional to the number of red blood cells moving together at nearly the same velocity. In this way, both the component frequencies and their amplitudes express the amount of flow organization within a sample volume inside a vascular compartment.

Through the Doppler equation, these frequency components become related to flow velocities. From these velocities come estimates of the amount of disease as well as volume blood flow within a vascular compartment or a heart chamber.

Volume flow, in turn, is a function of impediments to flow (flow resistance) and the driving energy delivered to the system. And in the end, viscosity-dependent energy loses will determine blood velocity. These energy losses will also affect the momentum of the moving blood, changing time relationship between a driving energy cycle (pulse pressure) and the blood flow response.[11]

Direction

The direction of flow within a vascular compartment and its changes over time can be used to detect flow disturbances. For example, in the heart, flow in the wrong direction can result from valve leakage or communicating defects within the cardiac septa that separate the heart's chambers. In the left vertebral artery, reversed flow indicates a subclavian steal. Direction also provides information about the presence of collateral flow in some vascular beds and whether or not an occlusion may be causing a major volume flow change in a vascular bed.[6]

The face of the transducer is the primary reference for direction. Flow logically separates into movement toward the transducer (forward flow) and movement away from the transducer (reverse flow). From the position of the transducer with respect to the vessel anatomy, direction can then be translated into flow direction within the vessel.

At times the direction of flow can appear paradoxical, especially if a sample volume includes only a small part of the overall pattern of flow within a vessel. For example, flow may be regionally reversing even though the overall flow is traveling down the vessel. Such regional reversals are subtle clues to flow disturbances along a vascular channel or through a cardiac valve.[10]

Common Ultrasound Problems

Doppler ultrasound may use transmitting techniques and echo-signal processing different from imaging ultrasound, but it is subject to the same problems of tissue-ultrasound interactions, such as tissue attenuation and poor acoustic reflectivity.

Once ultrasound is generated and echoes are formed, the primary problem is getting ultrasound to the target and an echo back to the transducer. This requires forming a beam, aiming it in the right direction, and choosing a frequency that permits adequate echo-signal return. This frequency choice may be crucial if the target is some distance within the tissues.

As the ultrasound burst travels to the target and returns, the tissue converts this organized mechanical energy into heat. In addition, small scattering bodies intercept the traveling ultrasound (both incident and echo) and scatter portions of the energy away. If a moving target is physically large and forms a specular reflection, then the strongest echo signals appear only when the beam is perpendicular to the target. If transducer or target movement points the beam off the perpendicular line, echo-signal strength falls off very rapidly.

In general, the echo signals that contribute to Doppler signal processing are from small scattering clusters of red blood cells, singular and in groups. The signal levels from these scattering sites are usually much smaller than the surrounding tissue signal levels. In fact, the tissue signals can be as much as 40 to 60 dB (100 to 1,000 times) larger than the smaller scattering-site signals.

The mix of very large signals from tissue interfaces and very small signals from blood scattering sites can make the process of extracting Doppler signals from the total mix very difficult.[12] The need to separate tissue from flow in the vicinity of vessel and heart chamber walls complicates signal processing.

Because the Doppler signals are of such small amplitude, resident noise in a system can quickly swamp these smallest of echo signals. Doppler sonographs often increase the overall output power of the transmitter to raise the echo signals above an internal noise floor. As a result, many Doppler systems have very high acoustic output powers. Noise also comes from the tissue in the form of nonstructural echoes, so-called, because they are not associated with any macroanatomy. Instead, they seem to come from interstitial tissue and functional tissue scattering sites within and surrounding organs and structures.[5] Such nonstructural echo signals are sensitive to the amount of tissue water, increasing in number and amplitude as the tissue water content decreases.

With this global view of Doppler ultrasound in hand, it is time to look at the associated events and signal processing in more detail.

References

1. O'Neill, WE, and Suga, N. Target range-sensitive neurons in the auditory cortex of the mustache bat. *Science* 203:69–73, 1979.
2. Creese, I, Burt, DR, and Snyder, SH. Proportionate tonotropic representation for processing CF-FM sonar signals in the mustache bat auditory cortex. *Science* 194:542–545, 1976.
3. Simmons, JA, Fenton, MB, and O'Farrell, MJ. Echolocation and pursuit of prey by bats. *Science* 203:16–21, 1979.
4. Griffin, DR. More about bat "radar". *In Animal Engineering.* San Francisco: W.H. Freeman, 1974, pp 73–77.
5. Powis, RL, and Powis, WJ. *A Thinker's Guide to Ultrasonic Imaging.* Baltimore: Urban & Schwarzenberg, 1984, pp 23–49, p 380.
6. Atkinson, P, and Woodcock, JP. *Doppler Ultrasound and Its Use in Clinical Measurement.* New York: Academic Press, 1982, pp 188–192.
7. Gosling, RG, and King, DH. Ultrasonic angiography. *In* Hascus, AW and Adamson, L (eds): *Arteries and Veins.* Edinburgh: Churchill Livingston, 1975, pp 61–98.
8. Thompson, RS, Trudinger, BJ, and Cook, CM. A comparison of Doppler ultrasound waveform indices in the umbilical artery—I. Indices derived from the maximum velocity waveform. *Ultrasound Med and Bio* 12:835–844, 1986.
9. Abdel-Azim, MS, and Hottinger, CF. *Multigate Doppler With Real Time Imaging for Blood Flow Analysis.* Technicare Ultrasound Technology Series, 1981.
10. Powis, RL. Angiodynography: A new real-time look at the vascular system. *Appl Radiol* 15:55–59, 1986.
11. Hatle, L, and Angelsen, B. *Doppler Ultrasound in Cardiology.* Philadelphia: Lea and Febiger, 1982, p 25.
12. Baker, DW, Forster, FK, and Daigle, RE. Doppler principles and techniques. *In* Fry, F J (ed): *Ultrasound: Its Applications in Medicine and Biology,* Part 1. New York: Elsevier Scientific, 1978, pp 161–287.

3

The Tissue–Ultrasound Interaction

As with processing for gray-scale imaging, Doppler depictions of flow are limited by the tissue–ultrasound interaction. Because this interaction plays such a central role in both applications, this chapter deals with its key events. The basic physical events within the tissue limit the use of Doppler ultrasound and help explain some of the differences between conventional echo ranging and Doppler signal processing. Events within the tissue also predict the design differences among the more advanced duplex imaging systems. The fundamental principles discussed here set the stage for tissue–ultrasound interactions that are the foundation of the balance of this book.

Ultrasound as a Mechanical Wave

Ultrasound is a mechanical, longitudinal wave, creating regional compressions and rarefactions of the carrying medium. Being mechanical, ultrasonic waves require something to carry them: a propagating medium; also known as a carrying material, or sometimes generically called tissue. Because the waves are mechanical, the physical characteristics of the medium define how the medium and waves interact.[1] This intimate contact between tissue and ultrasound provides an opportunity to use the interactions as a source of information about the tissue itself. The information, of course, resides in properties of the returning echo signals. Amplitude, for example, will become a gray-scale image, whereas phase and frequency components will be expressed as Doppler sounds.

Although ultrasound waves are mechanical, they still have the properties common to all waves. They are similar to electromagnetic waves, surface vibrations, and even transverse waves traveling down a string. In general, waves can add together in a simple manner, provided they are operating within the elastic limits of the carrying medium. Under these conditions, the original waves do not lose their individual identities. This wave property will be quite valuable when we begin to unravel events hidden in the summed waves of a Doppler signal.

A major aspect of the carrying medium or tissue is how fast the ultrasound moves through it. This is called the ultrasound velocity of propagation and is a constant at constant temperature. For most materials, the propagation velocity is also independent of the direction in which it is moving in the medium. Biological tissue can deviate from these two rules, however. The deviations are usually not large enough to introduce any serious errors, and the larger deviations such as bone are easy to identify.

The relationship between ultrasound wavelength and frequency is defined by the propagation velocity. When the propagation velocity is a constant, wavelength is determined by frequency. This relationship appears in the equation:

$$c = \lambda f \tag{3.1}$$

where c is the velocity of propagation in meters per second, λ is the wavelength in meters, and f is the frequency in hertz or cycles per second. This small equation simply states that if the velocity is constant, an increasing frequency produces a decreasing wavelength, and vice versa.

Our interest, however, should center on the wavelength portion of this equation. Many of the basic events in ultrasound such as reflection, attenuation, and even the Doppler effect depend upon the ultrasonic wavelength. A slight modification of the preceding equation will produce an easy calculation of wavelength for any ultrasound frequency:

$$1.54/f = \lambda \tag{3.2}$$

where f is in megahertz and λ is in millimeters. In other words, dividing the ultrasound frequency into 1.54 produces the ultrasonic wavelength; for example,

$$1.54/75 \text{ MHz} = 0.2 \text{ mm}$$

This relationship suggests that echo sources in the tissue smaller than 0.2 mm will reflect ultrasound differently from structures larger than 0.2 mm. The smaller structures become scattering bodies, and the larger structures become specular reflectors. The details of these two modes of reflection appear later in this discussion.

A major assumption when using ultrasound is that tissues in the body are isotropic, i.e., they have a constant velocity of propagation regardless of the direction in which the ultrasound moves in the tissue. This is a convenient assumption, but in reality, various tissues have propagation velocities that change with direction. Fortunately, most of these differences turn out to be relatively small. Table 3-1 shows the propagation velocities for several different tissues.

As ultrasound moves from one tissue region to another, small, local shifts in the propagation velocity change the wavelength. Thus, as an ultrasonic burst moves through the various tissues of the body, unpredictable but small variations in wavelength occur. For the remainder of this discussion, it is safe to consider the soft-tissue propagation velocity as a constant 1540 m/s, an assumption made by nearly every ultrasound machine.

Reflections at Interfaces

Reflections occur at acoustical interfaces within the tissue. An acoustical interface can be considered a plane where an abrupt change in acoustical impedance occurs. In practice, the interface can take on a wide range of complex shapes, but for now it is easier to understand the basic events in terms of a simple plane surface.

The mathematical definition of acoustic impedance (Z) is:

$$Z = \rho C \tag{3.3}$$

Table 3–1.   Ultrasound Propagation Velocities and Attenuation Rates

	m/s	*dB/cm/MHz*
Blood	1,549–1,565	0.18
Fat	1,476	0.63
Fat (eye)	1,582	
Liver (normal)	1,585	0.94
Liver (disease)	1,570	
Kidney	1,558–1,572	1.00
Spleen	1,570–1,578	
Connective tissue	1,545	
Skeletal muscle		
Longitudinal	1,592	1.30
Cross-sectional	1,545	3.30
Heart muscle	1,568–1,580	1.80
Neural tissue	1,524–1,540	
Bone	3,406–4,030	20.00
Skull	3,360	
Lung		41.00

where ρ is the mass density of the medium (g/cm³), and C is the ultrasonic velocity of propagation (cm/s). Clearly, a change in acoustic impedance at a reflecting interface can mean either a change in density, propagation velocity, or both.

In reality, very few of the acoustic interfaces in the body are perfect or nearly perfect reflectors. Most reflect poorly, returning only a fraction of a percent of the incident energy.

The amount of the incident energy reflected from any interface depends upon the change in acoustical impedance across that interface. A large change reflects more of the incident energy than an interface with a small change. Expressing this ability to reflect incident pressure waves is the reflection coefficient, *R:*

$$R = (Z_1 - Z_2)/(Z_1 + Z_2) \qquad (3.4)$$

where Z_1 and Z_2 are successive impedances encountered by an incident wave. In general, this equation states that the greater the impedance change at an interface, the greater the reflected energy. The energy not reflected continues on, encountering subsequent interfaces with reflections at each, until all the energy is finally reflected away or lost as heat in the tissue.

Reflection occurs in two different forms. The first is called specular reflection and follows the general rules of a mirror-like reflection. The second involves an interaction between the incident ultrasound and a very small reflecting body; this reflective process is called scattering.[2] Figure 3-1 illustrates these two forms of reflection.

Specular reflections generally occur at organ boundaries and tissue interfaces that have lateral dimensions greater than the wavelength of the incident ultrasound.[3] These include most organ capsules, the inner and outer walls of vessels, and plaque surfaces.

Specular reflection follows the rule that the angle of incidence is equal to the angle of reflection. Therefore, using specular reflections to see boundaries requires that the ultrasound beam be perpendicular to the interface. Figure 3-1 shows this geometric

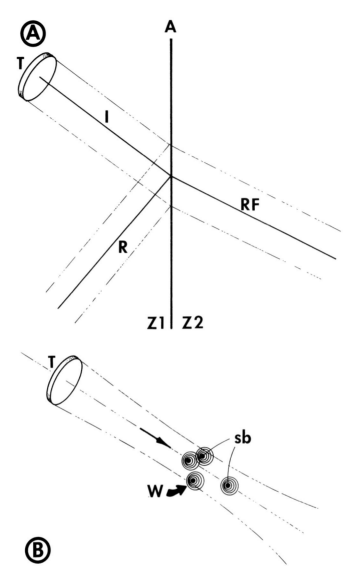

Figure 3-1   Ultrasonic reflections in the tissue. **A,** Specular reflections (*R*) occur at boundaries (*A*) where the acoustical impedance (*Z1, Z2*) changes. If the velocity of propagation changes, the ongoing ultrasound is refracted (*RF*). *I* is the incident beam, *T* is the transducer. **B,** The second form of reflection is scattering from small bodies (*sb*) that capture and reradiate the ultrasonic waves (*W*) in all directions.

rule. Although the amount of energy in the reflection may be constant, angling the beam away from 90° rapidly decreases the strength of the echo signal because less reflecting energy reaches the transducer (Fig. 3-2).

Scattering involves a physical interaction between the incident ultrasound and very small tissue structures. In general, these structures are smaller than the wavelength of the incident ultrasound.[2] Again, it is the lateral dimension of the scattering body and not the thickness of the interface that sets up this sort of reflection.

In ultrasound, scattering from isolated sites acts as if a portion of the incident ultrasonic energy were captured by the scattering body. The scattering body then re-

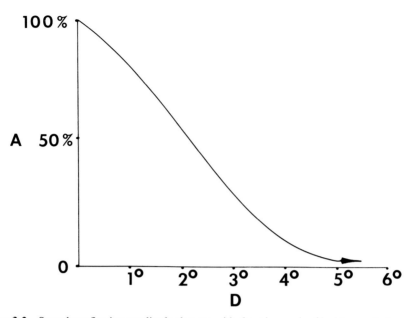

Figure 3-2   Specular reflection amplitude changes with changing angle of incidence. As the angle of incidence deviates (*D*) from 90°, the reflection amplitude (*A*) decreases.

radiates this energy in all directions.[2] As the reflected energy moves outward (Fig. 3-3), only a small portion of it reaches the transducer because of the spherical radiation pattern.

Scattering also can occur at specular interfaces where surface irregularities have sufficient dimension. If the surface roughness is very small with respect to the wavelength, scattering off these irregularities is small. But as roughness increases, the amount of scattering grows. As a consequence, we are often able to see the boundary of an organ or structure even though the transducer beam is not perpendicular to the surface.

An analogy to this sort of reflection is bouncing a ball off a flat floor that has stones spread over its surface. This is rather easy when the stones are very small. But if the stones should increase in size, the bouncing becomes more unpredictable as the ball

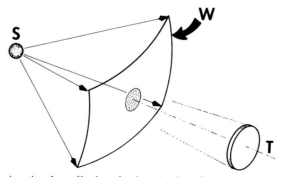

Figure 3-3   Scattering signal amplitude reduction. As the reflected wave (*W*) from a scattering site (*S*) expands from the local event, only a small portion (*shaded area*) actually reaches the transducer (*T*). As a result, scattering signals are typically very small.

is cast into different directions. In a similar manner, surface roughness on an acoustic interface can scatter ultrasound in a variety of directions

Because scattering casts energy in all directions, echoes from scattering bodies are much smaller than specular reflections from other tissue components. For the most part, the echo signals used for deriving Doppler information will come from scattering sites that are smaller than typical ultrasound wavelengths. The physical dimensions of these scattering sites range from about 7 to 50 μm.[4] In practice, these dimensions are the same for many tissue functional units, including human red blood cells, which individually and in clusters, act as effective scattering units.

Loss of Beam Energy

If ultrasound were to move through a medium with perfect elastic properties, the transfer of energy from one region of space to another would involve no energy losses. The movement of mechanical waves through biological tissue is not perfectly elastic, however. As a result, the waves alternately compress and pull apart the tissue inefficiently, converting a portion of the traveling wave energy into heat. This form of energy loss is called absorption.

Ultrasonic energy is also lost in scattering. As the microcomponents of tissue scatter the ultrasound away from the main beam, the ultrasonic energy spreads out. Only a portion of that spreading energy reaches the major targets on the way out and finally returns as an echo. The remaining energy is rescattered from surrounding tissue, which finally absorbs it. As a result, ultrasonic waves traveling through tissues with distributed scattering bodies steadily lose energy. This process differs from absorption in that the energy is not immediately converted into heat; instead, it simply spreads out from the travel waves and finally disappears into the thermal vibrations of the tissue's atoms and molecules.

The combination of these two mechanisms, absorption and scattering, form the overall process of attenuation. Because scattering and absorption are both frequency dependent, attenuation is also frequency dependent. In general, frequency-dependent attenuation is not linear for most tissues, but for the considerations and calculations here, assuming linearity is still very useful. Some typical frequency-dependent attenuation values for tissues and blood appear in Table 3-1.

Biological Conditions

Considering the significant histological variations in normal soft tissue, the range of biological specular reflectors within the body might also be great. This turns out to be a good logical extension. Strongly reflective interfaces in the body, for example, include bone–soft tissue and pericardium–lung interfaces. In contrast, weakly reflective interfaces include blood–brain, blood–kidney, blood–liver, and blood–soft plaque interfaces. Indeed, the ratio of these reflectivities from largest to smallest can easily exceed 100:1, which is a difference of 40 dB. Table 3-2 shows a collection of these various interfaces and their reflectivities compared to a perfect reflector that returns 100% of the incident energy. (Also see p. 33, "Deciphering the Decibel.")

The spread of reflective values for tissues in Table 3-2 shows a range of about 48 dB (a 250:1 ratio). This represents the dynamic range of specular tissue reflectivities. In

Table 3–2.   Tissue Reflectivities in Decibels Below a Perfect Reflector

Tissues	Z^a	Blood (1.61)	Bone (7.80)	Brain (1.58)	Fat (1.38)	Kidney (1.62)	Liver (1.65)	Muscle (1.70)	Water (1.48)	Soft tissue (1.63)
Air	0.00	0	0	0	0	0	0	0	0	0
Blood	1.61	*	−4	−41	−22	−50	−38	−31	−28	−44
Bone	7.80		*	−4	−3	−4	−4	−4	−3	−4
Brain	1.58			*	−23	−38	−33	−29	−30	−36
Fat	1.38				*	−22	−21	−20	−22	−22
Kidney	1.62					*	−41	−32	−50	−44
Liver	1.65						*	−37	−25	−44
Muscle	1.70							*	−23	−34
Water	1.48								*	−26
Soft tissue	1.63									*

^{a}Acoustic impedances (Z) in 10^{-5} g/cm²s.

An acoustic interface consists of two tissues with different acoustic impedences. Table 3-2 shows how the reflectivity (Eq. 3.4) of an interface changes with tissue changes on either side of the interface. Relative reflectivity is expressed in decibels below a perfect reflector (0 db). For example, a blood–kidney interface is −50 dB below a perfect reflector, which means that only 0.3% of the incident acoustic pressure wave reflects from the interface. In contrast, an air–kidney interface would be a perfect reflector, returning 100% of the incident acoustic pressure wave.

setting up an imaging sonograph, most of our effort will be to deliver this full range of echo signals to the image so that all the tissues can appear as gray scale on the screen.

Scattering from blood is found at the lower portion of this tissue reflectivity dynamic range. These small tissue signals also exhibit the so-called speckling effect from the transducer–tissue–ultrasound interaction. Speckling comes from the phase-dependent addition of echoes at the transducer.[5] It is the same sort of event that produces the sparkling in reflected laser light. The speckling phenomenon produces much of the texture we see in a gray-scale image. Because it depends upon the organization of the echo sources, speckle changes according to the histology of the various organs and tissues. Figure 3-4 shows the essential source of speckling and phase-sensitive detection in ultrasound.

As we noted earlier, blood reflections are at the lower end of the signal scale.[6] Large differences in reflectivity can create a frustrating situation of being able to depict tissues with imaging and yet being unable to obtain Doppler signals from vessels in the same region.

A complication in gathering Doppler information from blood is that ultrasound scattering is a function of hematocrit.[6] This function, however, is neither linear nor does it peak at hematocrit values typical of systemic blood (Fig. 3-5). The backscattering signal strength from blood reaches maximum at about a 20% hematocrit. It is almost linear in the 10% region, but steadily decreases in value beyond a 20%. Thus, normal hematocrits are located on the descending limb of this curve.

Although normal hematocrits are typically greater than 40%, chronically low values of 10% to 20% can be found in renal transplant patients on hemodialysis. Blood ultrasonic reflectivity will change markedly with rather small hematocrit swings in these patients.

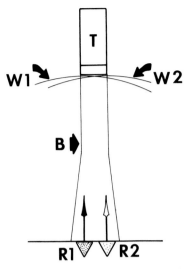

Figure 3-4   Phase-dependent wave reception at a transducer. In this experiment, reflecting bodies (*R1, R2*), simultaneously illuminated by the ultrasound beam (*B*), return two echoes 180° out of phase. These wave fronts (*W1, W2*) sum to zero at the transducer (*T*). Although large amounts of ultrasonic energy may be passing through the transducer, the two echo sources remain invisible to the imaging system. The superposition of waves makes this possible.

Measurements of blood acoustic properties suggest that the source of the Doppler echo signals is probably not individual red blood cells.[6] These cells are a lot smaller than a typical wavelength for ultrasound frequencies used in Doppler. For example, a red blood cell is 7 to 10 μm (7 × 10⁻⁶ m) in diameter, whereas a 10-MHz Doppler ultrasound wavelength is 0.154 mm (154 × 10⁻⁶ m), more than 20 times larger than a single red blood cell. With this sort of size difference, the backscattering from an indi-

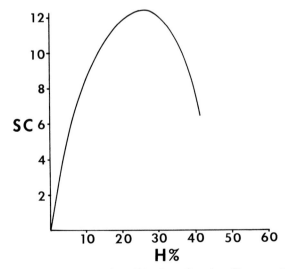

Figure 3-5   Effective scattering cross section of blood as a function of hematocrit. As the hematocrit (*H%*) increases from less than 10% to over 40%, the ability to backscatter ultrasound increases to a maximum near 25%, then decreases. This increase at 25% may represent the formation of effective scattering bodies in blood as aggregates of red blood cells.

vidual cell would be almost vanishingly small. Thus, aggregates of red blood cells are the real source of blood echo signals.

In fact, calculating backwards from the measured backscattering signal characteristics to a size estimate of the effective scattering unit in blood suggests that these sites are about 30 to 50 μm in diameter.[6] This corresponds closely to the size of scattering sites also found in solid, normal tissue.

In addition to scattering site size, distribution may also have an effect: blood may not fill a vascular compartment uniformly during systole or diastole. The Bernoulli principle (see Chapter 3) predicts, for example, that the higher velocity regions of blood flow will have a lower pressure. The pressure gradient between slower blood at a vessel edge and faster blood in the center results in red blood cell migration to the central lower pressure region. In support of this process are observations that red cell packing is at a maximum in the higher velocity regions of a vascular compartment.[7] This sort of vascular phenomenon occurs in both medium and small vessels.[7]

Clearly, regional changes in hematocrit can and will affect the reflectivity of blood. Furthermore, such changes will affect the ability to obtain Doppler information from some vascular compartments.

Reflection, Attenuation, and Penetration

Considering either tissue attenuation or the range of tissue reflectivities alone is not sufficient to establish realistic expectations about Doppler system performance. Combining these processes into a single model and diagram, however, could illustrate their effects and allow us to make some predictions about system performance and penetration.

To build this model, let us first observe a perfect reflector placed within an attenuating medium. In our example, the medium attenuation rate will be 1 dB/cm/MHz. A small thought experiment will reveal how this attenuation affects an echo and the resulting electronic echo signal: we will move the perfect reflector an increasing distance from the transducer within the uniform attenuating medium. The experimental result will be a graph of the received electrical signal amplitude as a function of the target range or distance from the transducer. Figure 3-6 illustrates the arrangement.

The reference for comparison will be 0 dB, the largest possible echo signal from the transducer, and the traditional way of expressing the reference level for decibel calculations. Obviously, this maximum signal occurs when the reflector is right in front of the transducer.

Moving the perfect reflector from in front of the transducer outward steadily decreases the echo-signal amplitude. If the smallest reflected signal our hypothetical imager can process is −100 dB below the reference (1/100,000th the largest signal), then signals falling below this lower limit will not appear. In this experiment, moving the reflector from the transducer face steadily reduces the echo-signal amplitude until it reaches the −100 dB level, where it vanishes from the display. This distance represents the maximum penetration for the system, even with a reflector returning 100% of the incident ultrasound. These results are shown in Figure 3-7.

The experiment will now be repeated with a less than perfect reflector, without changing the transducer output power. Now the starting echo signal at zero range will be lower than the 0-dB level. The attenuation rate remains the same, however, and the slope of this signal line parallels the perfect reflector line. Significantly, it not only starts at a lower value, but also vanishes earlier (Fig. 3-8). In general, then, echo sig-

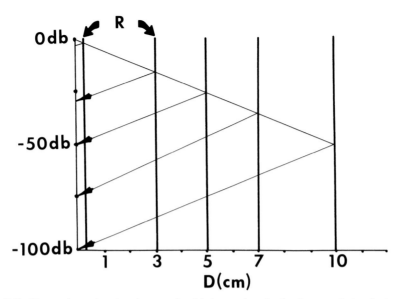

Figure 3-6   Decreasing echo signal strength with increasing depth. As a perfect reflector (*R*) is moved farther from a transducer (*D*) within an attenuating medium, the echo signal steadily decreases. When the signal amplitude falls below the lower limit (− 100 dB) of the system input dynamic range, the echo signal disappears. 0 dB represents the largest unsaturated input signal.

nals from smaller reflectors vanish earlier in an image than those from stronger reflectors. In application, this simple experiment shows why less reflecting interfaces vanish earlier than stronger ones in an ultrasound image.

Restoring penetration to a less reflective interface requires increasing the power from the transducer until the returning echo signal reaches the 0-dB level. In this new position, the echo signals from the interface vanish at the same depth as the perfect

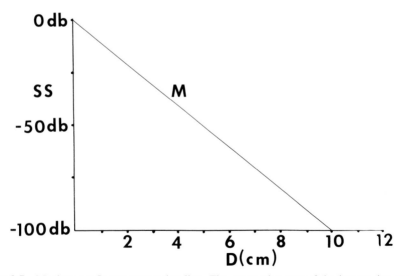

Figure 3-7   Maximum reflector attenuation line. The attenuation rate of the intervening material defines a maximum reflector attenuation line (*M*) that shows how deep into the medium this reflector can be seen. *D* is the target range; *SS* is the signal strength. At 10 cm, this example reflector vanishes from the screen.

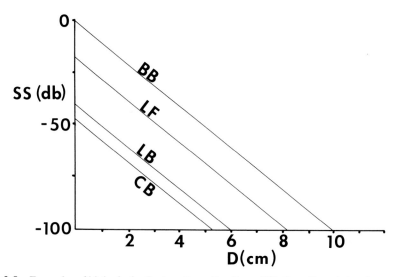

Figure 3-8   Examples of biological reflector attenuation lines. *SS* is the reflected signal strength and *D* is the range from the transducer. The maximum reflector is the blood-bone (*BB*) interface, which is typically less than 3 dB below a perfect reflector. *LF* is liver-fat, *LB* is liver-blood, and *CB* is the blood-brain interface, nearly 50 dB below the largest reflector.

reflector. This experiment not only demonstrates the rules governing effective penetration into tissue, but also the use of the system power control. A system power control is clearly different from system gain. Altering the system output changes the echo-signal amplitudes that *return* to the transducer. In contrast, changing system gain only changes those signals that are *already* inside the system. For this reason, system output will always have a greater influence on penetration than system gain.

Simply replacing the perfect reflector in the experimental medium with a strong biological reflector, without changing any imaging parameters, moves the attenuation line downward. Moving this maximum signal line to the former perfect reflector position requires increasing the system output until this signal reaches the 0-dB amplitude at the transducer. Adding some typical reflectors that span the range of normal biological reflectivities produces a mix of signals that range over 100 dB. The largest signal follows the original perfect reflector attenuation line. The smallest signal starts smaller and vanishes early, paralleling the largest signal line. The difference among signals due to reflectance is about 48 dB. Figure 3-8 demonstrates a basic rule of ultrasonic imaging: the smaller the reflectance, the sooner the signal vanishes from the display.

From this diagram comes another prediction about the tissue echo signals. Starting at the vanishing point of the smallest signal and deeper, the dynamic range of the tissue signals steadily decreases. Finally, even the most reflecting interfaces vanish from the display.

Let's consider a Doppler echo signal located 40 dB to 60 dB below the largest specular reflector. Clearly, this Doppler signal will vanish right along with the smallest biological signals. With this model in mind, a typical ultrasound image can offer clues about effective penetration of a Doppler system, provided, of course, that both systems use essentially the same output power.

Electronic amplifiers, as a rule, cannot handle a signal range spanning 100,000:1 (100 dB) unless the signals are compressed. In both imaging and Doppler applications, this sort of signal compression can be generated by using time-gain compensation. The overall processing focuses only on signal changes that represent differences in tissue reflectivity. Let's look at how this occurs.

As discussed earlier, echoes close to the transducer are very loud. That same reflector deeper in the tissue has a smaller amplitude because of tissue attenuation as the ultrasound travels out and back. Despite these differences in signal amplitude for the same sort of reflector, our imaging goal will be to make like reflectors look alike in the image. That means the stronger signals closer to the transducer must be reduced. At the same time, the weaker signals at a greater distance must be increased in size. As it turns out, we can change the amplitude of any signal by changing the system gain. Quite simply, we will turn down the volume for the signals close to the transducer and steadily increase the volume as the signals arrive from deeper portions of the tissue.

Because this change in gain must happen very quickly (every 13 μs represents 1 cm of tissue range), the system changes the gain automatically. Thus, we will set up the system to compensate for the tissue attenuation by changing gain as a function of time. Hence, time-gain compensation or TGC.

This compensation is set up by changing system gain over time (depth) to just match the rate at which all the signals are decreasing in amplitude. TGC, then, decreases the total dynamic range of the entering signals without losing the dynamic range of tissue reflectivities. The portrayal of tissue reflectivities is complete out to the range at which the smallest echo signals just vanish. Figure 3-9 shows this application of TGC.

One way of thinking about TGC is to consider a small problem in illumination. We begin with a strip of gray paper that steadily changes in gray shade from nearly white at one end to dark gray at the other. If we want to photograph this strip so that all the shades of gray appear the same, we can do this by illuminating it unequally. We could position a light overhead to brightly illuminate the darker segment and shade the lighter grays. If the angle of illumination is set just right, the darker grays become lighter and

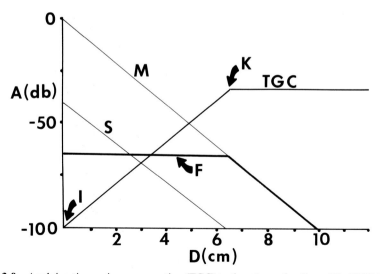

Figure 3-9   Applying time gain compensation (TGC) to the attenuation lines. The TGC is set up to increase gain from the initial (*I*) to the maximum (*K*) value at the same rate as tissue attenuation. As a result, the largest attenuation line (*M*) becomes a constant amplitude function (*F*) over the region of compensation. The smallest reflector attenuation line (*S*) sits 40 dB below *F*. *A* is signal amplitude, (*D*) is distance.

the lighter grays become darker. In this example, the gray strip represents the steady decrease in signal amplitude with depth; the illumination represents the system gain that shades the whiter grays and brightens the darker grays to make them appear to be the same intensity.

Correct adjustment of TGC for imaging, then, begins by setting the initial gain value so that the most and least reflective interfaces appear in the display dynamic range at the skin line. Then the TGC slope is set to maintain this signal dynamic range over the largest possible distance. Ideally, this would place the TGC knee at the vanishing point for the smallest signals. Within the image, all the strongest signals would be nearly white. The smallest signals from the scattering bodies would be a barely visible shade of gray. All the other reflectors would sit between these two gray scale limits. Beyond the knee, no compensation exists, and the echo-signal amplitudes and dynamic range decrease at a steady rate.

The information in the image depends upon displaying the full range of tissue reflectivities to depict differences among masses and tissues. Doppler, in turn, works with the smallest of these signals from some of the least reflecting objects, red blood cells. Attenuation rates and reflectivity combine to limit penetration and performance expectations for any Doppler system. From these physical events emerge some general rules: 1) tissue attenuation affects the small echoes in the same manner as large echoes; 2) the attenuation rate and the loss of information is frequency dependent, increasing with an increasing frequency; and 3) overall penetration decreases with increasing frequency.

Refraction Influences

Refraction is a process that displaces an ultrasonic beam from its normally straight propagation pathway as it moves through different tissues (Fig. 3-10). It occurs at inter-

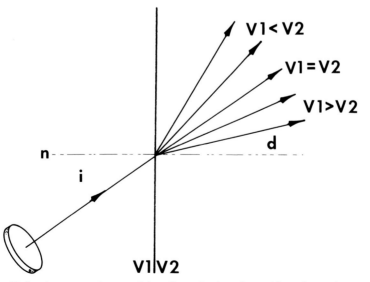

Figure 3-10   Refraction at an ultrasound interface. An interface with a change in propagation velocity (*V1, V2*) bends the ultrasound beam when the incident angle (*i*) is not 90°. *n* is the normal line, *d* is the deviation angle. With no velocity change, the beam remains unbent, i.e., *V1* = *V2*.

faces where the wave propagation velocity changes and the beam is not perpendicular to the interface. The refraction process is, in fact, expressed by an equation called Snell's law. This relationship includes both the angle of incidence to the interface and the change in velocity that deviates the traveling ultrasound pathway. Snell's law appears in equation form as

$$V_1/V_2 = (\sin i)/(\sin d) \tag{3.5}$$

where V is the propagation velocities in each of the materials, i is the incident angle, and d is the deviation angle.

The rules for ultrasonic refraction in tissue are the same as for light moving through air and water. Looking at a fish in a pool of water is a bit illusory because the fish is not actually located where its image suggests. The light reflecting from the fish refracts at the air–water interface. Thus, a spear fisherman knows he must aim under the image of the fish to finally spear it; if he aims at the fish, the spear will miss.

Scanning a vessel in cross section often creates shadows extending down from the vessel walls. These shadows come from the refraction of ultrasound inside the vessel walls.[8] In addition, refraction at the boundary of a cystic structure can cast a shadow over a nearby vessel wall. Such a shadow could be confused with a shadowing plaque rather than refraction at the cyst wall.

Refraction can also occur at boundaries that are physically shaped into a natural lens; one good source is skeletal muscle. The muscle and its surrounding sheath provide both a change in wave velocity and a lens shape in cross section.[9] One result of such a lens formation is the "double uterus" artifact that appears as ultrasound refracts through the abdominal muscles.[9] Other well-formed muscle groups such as the sternocleidomastoideus have a similar potential for lensing effects (Fig. 3-11).

Artifacts from the Tissue–Ultrasound Interaction

A common and obvious artifact that appears in ultrasound is reverberations. These signal patterns can arise anywhere within an image from two highly reflective interfaces that are physically parallel to one another and mutually perpendicular to the ultrasound beam axis. Figure 3-12 is a schematic of this geometric condition and an image example of the phenomenon.

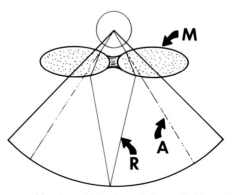

Figure 3-11   Lens effects caused by shaped interfaces. Masses that have shapes like lenses (*M*) and also have differing propagation velocities can bend beams (*R*) away from expected paths (*A*). Such masses include soft tissues such as muscles or fatty tumors. Scanning through the abdominus rectus muscles often produces double uteruses in some images of the lower abdomen.

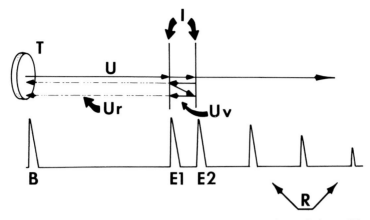

Figure 3-12   Ultrasound reverberation in the tissues. An incident ultrasonic beam (*U*) can end up reverberating (*Uv*) between two strong reflectors (*I*) to create reverberation signals (*R*). On each bounce, some of the ultrasound (*Ur*) leaks back to the transducer, *T* is the transducer, *B* is the transmit signal, and *E1* and *E2* are primary echo signals from the interfaces.

Frequently, one of the two interfaces is the transducer–skin contact surface, while another deeper structure creates a second reflecting surface. In this situation, the reverberation extends right from the skin surface deeply into the image. A common source of deeper reverberations is calcified soft tissue, which forms surfaces parallel and close to one another, and at the same time, perpendicular to the ultrasound beam. In the abdomen, a very common source is the air–soft tissue interface. Long reverberations often extend from pockets of bowel gas mixed with food traveling through the gastrointestinal tract.

Typically, reverberations appear in the image as a series of evenly spaced echo signals that extend into the image from the first reverberation surface. Tissue attenuation and transmission through both interfaces steadily decreases the reverberation amplitude over time. Unfortunately, reverberations often have amplitudes large enough to hide smaller echo signals within the tissue image. This can be especially troublesome for Doppler signal processing because of its dependence upon small signals. If the reverberation produces changes in the phase or timing of the returning echo signal, it can confuse the Doppler signal processing.

Another highly visible artifact is acoustical shadowing that results from very attenuating materials or very reflective interfaces (Fig. 3-13, see color section between pp. 116 and 117). The shadows begin at the intervening structures that absorb or reflect the ultrasound and extend into the image. Shadowing affects the ability to see deeper structures by lowering the strength of the echo signals returning from structures within the shadows or by eliminating ultrasound propagation entirely. Thus, signals from deeper structures can be absent from the final image.

Loss of signal strength with shadowing can drastically affect Doppler processing, reducing or completely eliminating recovery of effective signals from within the shadow. Doppler is already pivoting on the smallest echo signals, so even mild shadowing can have a major effect.

Importantly, a shadowing mass is not always calcified tissue. Masses, including plaques, that are highly fibrotic can also shadow without producing strong echo signals from the primary structure. Shadows can also appear in quite normal tissue. These absorption shadows often appear in the tissues of young, normal people.

Shadowing lesions seldom completely surround a vascular compartment, so

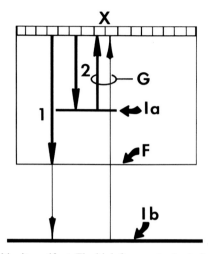

Figure 3-14   The range ambiguity artifact. The high frame rates typical of current real-time systems can generate a range ambiguity artifact. In this sequence, the transducer array (*X*) sends out an ultrasound burst (*1*). The burst continues beyond the field of view (*F*) to a distant reflector (*Ib*). During the subsequent pulse-listen cycle (*2*), echoes from the distant source (*Ib*) arrive at the transducer at the same time (*G*) as echoes from a more proximal echo source (*Ia*). The artifact is the appearance of structure *Ib* at the image position of *Ia*.

changing the scanning position is one way of viewing flow hidden in the primary image. New scanning positions, however, can be difficult to sort out for a reader unfamiliar with the approach. Including a vascular landmark can do a lot to improve the understanding of an image and its associated Doppler spectrum.

One of the most insidious sources of shadowing is an inadequate coupling between the transducer and the skin surface. Coupling gel that has air bubbles or simply the lack of gel at the transducer–skin interface can destroy an otherwise excellent scan. The solutions to this problem are easy: 1) use lots of scanning gel; and 2) renew the gel frequently.

In a stable, unmoving image, shadows that reduce signals by 3 dB to 6 dB can be hard to see. Moving a real time scanhead and watching the changing image often brings out even the most subtle shadow. These shadows are not only clues to the character of the tissues surrounding a vessel, but also provide hints that a new transducer position many be needed to avoid weak Doppler signals.

A subtle and almost mysterious form of artifact is the arrival at the transducer of echo signals that came from earlier pulse-listen cycles.[10] These signals form what is called the range ambiguity artifact (Fig. 3-14). This artifact also has a variety of more descriptive names such as "Herbie" and "ring around artifact." Range ambiguity artifacts are a problem because they can create the illusion of masses or structures where none exist.

This artifact comes from the contemporary requirements of high frame rates in real-time systems. Early real-time systems had few scan lines and low frame rates; thus, each pulse-listen cycle had time to die out before the next pulse-listen cycle occurred. As a result, echoes from deep structures outside the image depth were allowed to die out. Our current imaging procedures, however, require higher frame rates and pulse repetition frequencies. As a result, the system generates the next pulse-listen cycle before all the echoes from the previous cycle have died out. The range ambiguity comes from the fact that the echoes from the deeper structures appear closer to the transducer than they really are.

In general, an ultrasound system operates at a steady pulse repetition frequency (PRF) in any operating mode. This makes the system particularly sensitive to echo signals from deeper structures or from reverberations that temporally resonate with the pulse repetition frequency. One way of testing for these time-dependent artifacts is to shift the system PRF or the image frame rate (effectively changing the PRF). This test works if the system frame rate is a function of the field of view, and if altering the display depth changes the PRF. When the PRF changes, range ambiguity artifacts will either change position in the image or vanish completely.

The range ambiguity artifact depends entirely on the time relationship between the system PRF and the location of the deeper echo source. Changing this time relationship, of course, changes the position or appearance of the artifact. As we noted earlier, changing the PRF will move the artifact. Alternately, the sonographer may be able to change the position of the echo source. The range ambiguity artifact in neonatal head scanning, for example, often comes from the skin–air interface as the scanhead points toward the occipital portion of the baby's head. If the sonographer puts a hand on the baby's head in this location, the artifact will move. A range ambiguity artifact can also appear when scanning large cystic structures such as a testicular hydrocele. Again, if the sonographer's hand on the posterior surface causes the entity to move, that movement clearly identifies it as an artifact.

Interestingly, some Doppler signal-processing systems will use the range ambiguity process to handle higher Doppler shift frequencies without aliasing. The exact features of this technique are covered in Chapter 8.

To reiterate, ultrasound is a mechanical wave that must be carried by a medium, which is soft tissue in our application here. There are two basic interactions between ultrasound and the tissue. First, the ultrasound acts upon the tissue through compression, rarefaction, and the direct heating of the tissue. Second, the tissue acts on the ultrasound, causing a loss of energy through scattering and absorption. Each of the interfaces in the tissue that has a change in acoustic impedance generates an echo, sometimes large, sometimes small. Ultimately, it is the sum of all the tissue–ultrasound effects that generates the final image and influences our perception of the anatomy and physiology that the image portrays.

Deciphering the Decibel

After the Hertz, the decibel is probably the most used unit in ultrasound—and the least understood. In the end, the decibel is only a ratio of values with one being a reference value. It is a way of handling large, otherwise cumbersome numbers in a shorthand way by expressing the ratios as logarithms. Two equations exist: one for voltage and amplitudes, another for power and energy. The voltage form is:

$$dB = 20 \, Log \, (V/R)$$

and the power form is:

$$dB = 10 \, Log \, (P/R)$$

where dB is the decibel value, Log is the base 10 logarithm, V is a measured voltage, P is a measured power, and R is the reference value.

Logarithms are exponents, which means a logarithm of a number is the power to which 10 would be raised to obtain that number. For example, the Log of a 1000:1 ratio is 3 ($10^3 = 1000$).

For *voltage* ratios, then, a 1000:1 is $20 \times 3 = 60$ dB, 100:1 is $20 \times 2 = 40$ dB, and 2:1 is $20 \times 0.3 = 6$ dB.

For *power* ratios, 1000:1 is $10 \times 3 = 30$ dB, 100:1 is $10 \times 2 = 20$ dB, and 2:1 is $10 \times 0.3 = 3$ dB.

On a more practical basis, manufacturers often express system gain levels in dB as a voltage ratio. Thus, increasing system gain by 6 dB doubles internal echo signal amplitudes; taking the system gain down 6 dB reduces them by one half.

References

1. Nyborg, WL. Principles of ultrasound. *In* Fry FJ (ed): *Ultrasound: Its Applications in Medicine and Biology.* New York: Elsevier Scientific, 1978, pp 1–76.
2. Nicholas, D. An introduction to the theory of acoustic scattering by biological tissues. *In* White DN (ed): *Recent Advances in Ultrasound in Biomedicine.* Forest Grove, OR: Research Studies Press, 1977, pp 1–28.
3. Edmonds, PD, and Dunn, F. Introduction: Physical description of ultrasonic fields. *In* Edmonds PD (ed): *Methods of Experimental Physics,* vol 19, *Ultrasonics.* New York: Academic Press, 1981, pp 1–28.
4. Reid, JM, and Shung, KK. Quantitative measurements of scattering of ultrasound by heart and liver. *In* Linzer M. (ed): *Ultrasonic Tissue Characterization II,* National Bureau of Standards Special Publication 525. Washington, DC: US Government Printing Office, 1979, pp 153–156.
5. Burckhardt, CB. Speckle in ultrasound B-mode scans. *IEEE Transactions on Sonics and Ultrasonics,* SU-25 (1):1–6, 1978.
6. Hanss, M, and Boynard, M. Ultrasound backscattering from blood: Hematocrit and erythrocyte aggregation dependence. *In* Linzer M (ed): *Ultrasonic Tissue Characterization II,* National Bureau of Standards Special Publication 525. Washington, DC: US Government Printing Office, 1979, pp 165–169.
7. Ganong, WF. *Review of Medical Physiology.* Los Altos, CA: Lange Medical, 1969, p 463.
8. McDicken, WN. *Diagnostic Ultrasonics: Principles and Use of Instruments,* ed 2. New York: John Wiley and Sons, 1981, p 63.
9. Muller, N, Cooperberg, PL, Rowley, VA, et al. Ultrasonic refraction by the rectus abdominis: The double image artifact. *J Ultrasound Med* 3:515–519, 1984.
10. Goldstein, A. Range ambiguities in real-time ultrasound. *J Clin Ultrasound* 9:83–90, 1981.

4

Building a Model of Blood Flow

Purpose and Direction

Before any of the sounds, spectral recordings, or flow mapping used in Doppler ultrasound can make any sense, we have to understand something about how blood moves within vessels and heart chambers. Understanding blood flow in health, of course, sets the stage for detecting disease and often assessing the character and extent of the disease process. In turn, picturing the fluid properties of blood rests on understanding the properties of fluids in general. These properties provide a coherent view of how blood moves and some expectations for its behavior within the cardiovascular system.

This discussion starts with stationary fluids (statics), then proceeds to moving fluids (dynamics), and ends with a close look at some of the known behavior of blood as a moving fluid (hemodynamics). Both the fluidics of blood developed in this chapter and the blood–ultrasound interaction discussed in Chapter 3 are central to the examination of Doppler signal processing in later chapters.

How much of the theory of fluids do we need to understand hemodynamics and the clinical applications of Doppler ultrasound? Volumes have been written on the mathematical description of fluids at rest and in motion.[1] We certainly do not need such a heavily mathematical approach; nevertheless, some of the practical aspects of hydrostatics and hydrodynamics will be applicable to clinical medicine. The task is to strike a balance between the level of understanding necessary to use current Doppler ultrasound technology and a few of the more complex principles of fluids that are useful to appreciate some of the emerging clinical applications of Doppler. These new forms of Doppler will replace existing dangerous, invasive imaging procedures and open new windows for understanding the pathophysiology of disease.

Fluids at Rest: Hydrostatics

A fluid uncontained is a fluid out of control. It will spread everywhere, flowing downhill, freely expanding over flat surfaces, seeping through joints or fingers trying to hold it. How rapidly it moves depends upon a quality of the fluid we could call thickness: thin fluids move freely; thick fluids move slowly.

A fluid has no shape of its own, only that of the container holding it because it lacks internal rigidity. It has an internal structure, but that usually applies only at the atomic or molecular level. Still, fluids have forces that extend from molecule to molecule, trying to pull everything together. These forces are not very strong, which gives meaning to our concept of what constitutes a fluid.

Water is a good example of a fluid that completely conforms to the minute variations in the shape of its container. It was this chameleon-like quality of water that created the first fluid paradox in hydrostatics. This paradox emerges when a complex container with many differently shaped openings is filled with water (Fig. 4-1). As water pours into the container, it conforms to each of the shapes, eventually reaching equilibrium. At equilibrium, the water level in each of the different openings is the same. This forms the paradox. What keeps the obviously larger weights of water contained in the larger shapes from pushing out the narrow columns of water? The properties of fluids that emerge from this discussion explain how the paradox occurs.

At the outset, water flows downhill because it has mass and responds to the earth's gravitational field. As a result, a container holding water has a weight determined by the volume of water within it (Fig. 4-2). The mass of the water is expressed as mass density in units of mass per unit volume such as grams per cubic millimeter. The force exerted on each unit volume of a fluid is determined by Newton's second law, which states that force is the product of the mass density times the gravitational acceleration, g. A cubic centimeter of fluid, for example, will have a weight determined by this multiplication of mass density by g.

To determine the pressure exerted on the bottom of a cube by its weight, we divide the weight (force) by the area of the cube bottom. Determining the pressure caused by a column of fluid, then, requires adding up all the vertical cubes. In a generalized form, the result is the hydrostatic pressure (P) equation:

$$P = -pgh \qquad (4.1)$$

where p is the mass density of the fluid, g is the gravitational accelerations, and h is the height of the fluid within the gravitational field. In other words, at the top of a container

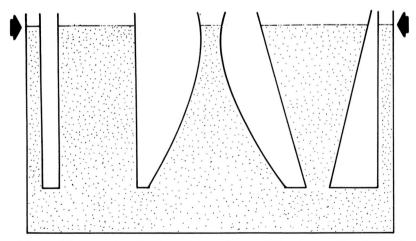

Figure 4-1   First fluid paradox. In this container of many different connecting shapes, the large masses of water do not push out the smaller masses. Why? Pressure along the bottom connection is constant regardless of the shape of the container above, therefore, all continuous water columns have the same height (*arrows*). The observation: water seeks its own level.

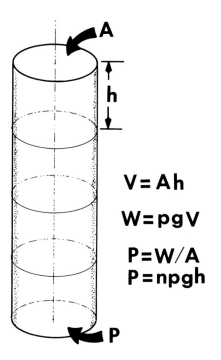

$$V = Ah$$

$$W = pgV$$

$$P = W/A$$

$$P = npgh$$

Figure 4-2 Pressure from a fluid column. A fluid column can be thought of as a set of smaller water volumes (*V*) with a height (*h*) and an area (*A*). A unit weight (*W*) is the product of the mass density of the fluid (*p*), gravitational acceleration (*g*), and the unit volume (*V*). Pressure (*P*) is weight (*W*) per unit area (*A*), so the hydrostatic pressure (*P*) is the sum (*n*) of all the small height changes (*h*) times mass density (*p*) and gravitational acceleration (*g*).

of water, the hydrostatic pressure is zero, and grows directly with depth in the fluid.

Measuring pressures horizontally shows that the hydrostatic pressure is constant along any horizontal line. But does this mean that the pressure only applies to the vertical direction? A pressure transducer pointing in any direction from a single point within a fluid, however, will read the same pressure. In other words, a particle of fluid feels the same pressure from all sides. Hydrostatic pressure in a fluid is clearly independent of direction.

A change in shape makes no difference, either. In a container, regardless of shape, the pressure along a horizontal line is constant, dependent only on the vertical distance from the top of the fluid. From these observations comes a primary law of hydrostatics: pressure at any point in a fluid is independent of direction and depends only on the depth of the point within the fluid.[2] The answer to the first hydrostatic paradox, then, is that the pressure exerted by a thin column or a large column or a strangely shaped column is the same. This brings the fluid to equilibrium in complex, connected containers as well as in a single, simple container.

This first law of hydrostatics has some conditions, however. First, the fluid surface must be free of any external pressure. Second, the fluid must be incompressible. This means that applying pressure to the fluid does not force the fluid molecules closer together, producing a change in the fluid density.

Hydrostatic principles also apply to the physiology of normal venous circulation in the lower extremities. In an upright man, at rest, the venous system resembles the previously described, complex container. The venous pressure in the tibial veins at the ankle, in the absence of active muscle contraction, can be calculated from basic principles: the mass (specific gravity) of blood, which is 1.056 g/cm³, times the gravitational acceleration (980 cm/s²) times the column height of blood from ankle to heart gives the pressure. Thus, the venous pressure in the ankle vein of a healthy man 70 in. (178 cm) tall is about 100 mmHg. In the normal venous system, active muscle contraction and venous valves to overcome this hydrostatic pressure and blood returns to the heart. Diseases that impair venous return to the heart produce high venous ankle pressures as part of the pathophysiology.

Despite the rather uncomplicated qualities of hydrostatics up to now, we have not exhausted all the available paradoxes. One remains, suggested by the experience of moving fluids through pipes. In simple terms, a fluid will move through a pipe if we apply pressure to one end and open the other. The fluid moves because a pressure gradient exists between the pressure end of the pipe and the open end. Fluids, it seems, move down pressure gradients.

Surprisingly, an open container filled with a fluid will produce a very similar situation. If we start measuring pressures within the standing fluid, the following situation emerges: measurements at the surface will equal the atmospheric pressure; at some distance into the fluid, the pressure will be higher than the surface; and at the bottom of the container sits the highest pressure. Indeed, this pressure is predicted by the hydrostatic equation (Fig. 4-3). If the top of the fluid has the lowest hydrostatic pressure and the bottom the highest, what then prevents the fluid from flowing along this pressure gradient and out of the flask? The answer to this paradox arrives later in the discussion on moving fluids.

Applying an external pressure to a contained fluid and observing the results generalizes the hydrostatics rule a bit more. Figure 4-4 shows the new conditions of this experiment. A piston now presses down on the fluid surface, exerting a pressure. Measurements inside the fluid show that at any point, the absolute pressure (P_{abs}) will be the sum of the external pressure and the internal hydrostatic pressure, that is,

$$P_{abs} = P_{ext} + pgh \qquad (4.2)$$

where P_{ext} is the external pressure. Regardless of where the pressure is measured in the fluid, this condition is true. Indeed, it seems that pressure applied to a fluid by any method is felt throughout the fluid, undiminished by distance or the general character of the pressure.[2] This uniform, unencumbered transmission of pressure through a fluid is called *Pascal's law* and is a central property of fluids, whether moving or not.

This property of undiminished pressure transmission in a fluid can be harnessed to obtain a gain in force, as if the fluid were a liquid lever. Figure 4-5 shows the new conditions for this hydrostatic situation: a container of fluid between two pistons of different sizes. The gain in force is based on the relationship that pressure is equal to force per unit area.

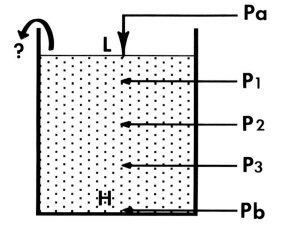

Figure 4-3 Second fluid paradox. Pressure measurements in a fluid filled flask show a set of increasing pressures. *Pa* is the atmospheric pressure, *Pa* < *P1* < *P2* < *P3* < *Pb*, where *Pb* is the bottom pressure. If pressure moves fluids, what keeps the fluid in the flask, despite the difference in pressure between *H* and *L*?

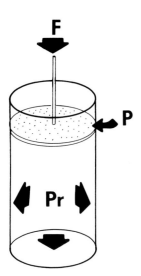

Figure 4-4 Fluid distribution of pressure. Applying a force (*F*) to the piston (*P*) exerts a pressure throughout the fluid (*Pr*). This even distribution of applied pressure throughout a fluid is part of Pascal's law of fluids.

Applying force to the smaller piston produces an increase in pressure equal to the applied force divided by the area of that piston. At the same time, the larger piston experiences that very same pressure. Because it has a larger area, however, the rod on piston B will receive a much larger force. The actual gain is proportional to the ratio of the two piston areas. On a practical basis, this arrangement can brake a car or lift heavy weights. More to the point for our discussion, this fluid gain in force will change the behavior of pressure waves traveling from a beating heart through the many vessels of the cardiovascular system to produce a pulse at the distal portion of an extremity.

A good question to ask at this point in the discussion is: How fast do pressure changes move within in a fluid? Is a pressure change instantaneously transmitted or does it take time? Measurements show that a pressure wave moves very quickly but not instantaneously through a fluid. Mathematical calculations and direct observations indicate that pressure moves through a fluid at the acoustic propagation velocity of the fluid.[2] In water, it is about 1,480 m/s; in blood, about 1,580 m/s.

But if pressure can move so quickly through a fluid, why does it take so long for the beat of a heart to arrive as a pulse in a peripheral artery? Measurements show that pulse waves move at 5 to 10 m/s in the vascular system, not 1,580 m/s.[3] The source of this difference becomes apparent from the nature of the fluid container, the vessels themselves.

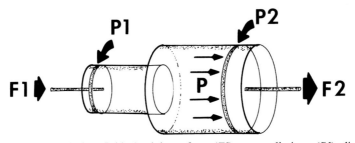

Figure 4-5 Hydraulic gain in a fluid. Applying a force (*F1*) to a small piston (*P1*), distributes the pressure (*P*) throughout the fluid, including the much larger second piston (*P2*). The larger surface area of the second piston gathers more pressure energy, which produces a larger force (*F2*) from the second piston.

Pressure propagation measurements usually take place in a rigid compartment with walls that do not change dimension with changing pressure. In contrast, the pulse pressure in the vascular system travels along flexible pipes that propagate the pressure wave slowly, using a surface wave that deforms the vessel wall.[4] Therefore, the solution to this paradox of pressure and pulse propagation lies in the distensibility of the vessel walls.

In summary, some thought experiments and a few common human experiences with fluids have revealed some basic properties of fluids at rest: 1) fluids have mass and respond to a gravitational field; 2) fluids are incompressible, or at least considered so; 3) pressures move through fluids at sonic propagation velocities if the container is rigid, but move at a slower velocity in compliant blood vessels; 4) pressure at a point in a fluid is the same in all directions (Pascal's law); and 5) some hydraulic principles can be applied to provide a force gain through a fluid-pressure system. Fluids in motion show all of these properties and a few more, which will be explained as our discussion unfolds.

Fluids in Motion: Hydrodynamics

Pouring a fluid out of a container releases it to follow its unconfined nature. As it moves from the edge of the container into the air, the fluid changes shape, revealing some of its internal forces. Along with the shape change, the fluid fails to fall straight down from the edge of the container. Instead, it arcs outward as the inertia from the forward motion carries the fluid into space. Fluids that have mass and are in motion carry inertia in each unit volume. Free in space, the forces among the fluid molecules shape the liquid stream into a cascading cylinder. Fluids in space (zero gravitation) collapse into spheres in response to these same forces.

If we could put a small spot of ink in the fluid just before we pour it out, that spot would move and inscribe an arc in space. The arc represents the motion of a single fluid particle. This line of motion is smooth and continuous (Fig. 4-6), and represents one of the more effective analytical tools for hydrodynamics, the streamline.[5]

The streamline in fluid dynamics is like ray formation in optics. It provides a means of following what would be otherwise hard to visualize. Along the streamline, we can consider continuity of motion, energy, and momentum, all valuable in understanding the motion of fluids. This streamline formation, originally just the domain of the hydrodynamicist, is a recognizable event in the vascular system of humans. Clinicians are beginning to recognize that alterations of the streamline formations in flowing blood can characterize disease states in vessels such as the carotid arteries.

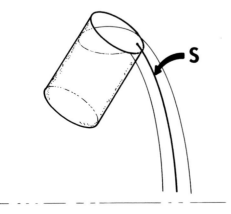

Figure 4-6 Pouring fluid streamline. Putting a drop of ink in a fluid and then pouring it shows how the fluid moves. In this case, the dot would inscribe a continuous arc (*S*). This unbroken motion of fluid particles defines a streamline.

Moving Fluids Through Pipes: A Look at Volume Flow

A first question to ask about a fluid moving through any pipe is: How much fluid is actually going through the pipe? This question can be answered two ways, in terms of the volume of material moving along during each unit of time or the velocity of the fluid within the pipe. The first approach uses the concept of volume flow, which has units of volume per unit time. For vessels it could be milliliters per second; for cardiac output, liters per minute. The second approach uses the speed (velocity) of the moving fluid and has units of distance per unit time. In peripheral vessels, it is expressed as centimeters per second. But these two views of flow, volume and velocity are not so far apart. Volume flow (Q) is a function of the pipe cross-sectional area (A) times the spatial average fluid velocity (V), that is:

$$Q = VA \tag{4.3}$$

Some of the assumptions and rules governing this equation will be more easily seen if we look at the piston model, as shown in Figure 4-7.

The double piston model uses a constant diameter pipe with pistons at each end. Pushing one piston in makes the other move out. The volume pushed in by the first piston can be calculated by

$$V_1 = A\, d_1 \tag{4.4}$$

where V_1 is the volume, A is the cross-sectional area, and d_1 is the displacement distance. Following the same rule, the volume displaced by the second piston is

$$V_2 = A\, d_2 \tag{4.5}$$

These two volumes are equal if the fluid involved is incompressible, and the walls of the pipe do not change shape. The equality of these volumes comes from the conservation of mass and fluid incompressibility. The conservation of mass simply means that the process did not destroy or create mass. In other words, what goes into the pipe must come out the other side.

Moving piston 1 over a specific time interval (dt) permits relating distance and time. Dividing both sides of the volume equation by dt produces

$$V_1/dt = A\,(d_1/dt) \tag{4.6}$$

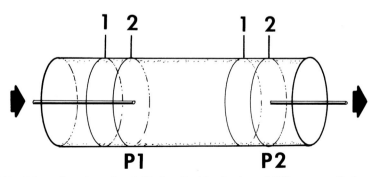

Figure 4-7   Volume flow through a rigid pipe. Pushing in piston 1 (*P1*) causes a displacement from position *1* to *2*. The second piston (*P2*) moves out, covering the same distance (*1* to *2*) if the areas are the same. This holds true only if the fluid is incompressible and the conservation of mass applies.

where V_1/dt is volume per unit time and d_1/dt is velocity v_1 (length per unit time). This equation reduces to

$$Q = A\,v_1 \qquad\qquad (4.7)$$

which is our original volume flow, area, and velocity relationship, with a strong assumption that what goes in must come out.

Displacing piston 1 means delivering a force to the piston, which, in turn, exerts a pressure on the fluid within the pipe. Plotting the driving pressure versus the volume flow in a pipe is instructive when looking at flow mechanics (Fig. 4-8). From zero to a relatively large pressure, a linear relationship exists between pressure and volume flow. The slope of this line, which is the rate of change in volume flow with respect to a change in the applied pressure, is a constant. The pressure-volume relationship shown on the graph can be expressed in the following equation:

$$Q = P/R \qquad\qquad (4.8)$$

where P is the applied pressure, Q is the volume flow through the pipe, and R is the resistance of the pipe.

This relationship between pressure, volume flow, and resistance is called *Poiseuille's equation* (Jean Leonard Marie Poiseuille, 1797–1869). This equation can be used to answer the question of how much fluid is moving through a pipe. It is quite similar to Ohm's law for electronics, $I = E/R$, which relates the flow of current I, driven by a voltage E, through a resistance R. Poiseuille's equation will be valuable for determining volume flow through peripheral arteries and veins, and bypass grafts, as well as for evaluating cardiac output and stroke volume.

In the volume flow equation, pressure and volume flow are measurable. Right now, we know the least about the resistance term, and it deserves a closer look.

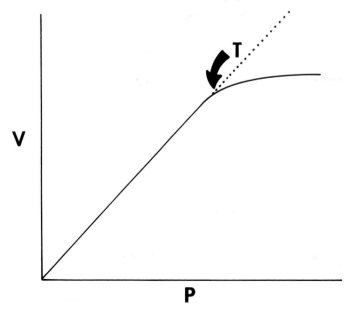

Figure 4-8   Volume flow as a function of applied pressure. Over a relatively wide range of values, pressure (P) and volume flow (V) are linearly related. As the fluid flow becomes unstable, however, increases in pressure do not produce a linear increase in volume flow (T). At this point, energy begins to go into supporting the complex fluid motion rather than increased volume flow.

Resistance to Flow

Trying to move a fluid through a pipe involves not only the physical properties of that fluid, but also an interaction between the pipe and the fluid. For example, as a pipe becomes longer, more fluid is in contact with the pipe walls, and it requires a higher pressure to maintain fluid movement. And, of course, if the fluid is thick, with a lot of internal forces between molecules, it will take more energy to move the fluid. This thickness property is fluid viscosity, and the forces are viscous forces.

Compared to viscous forces and pipe length, a change in the diameter of a pipe has an even more dramatic effect on resistance: the resistance changes with the radius to the fourth power. This effect, combined with the other two, provides the following equation for resistance:

$$R = 8\,nL/\,\pi\,r^4 \tag{4.9}$$

where R is the collective flow resistance, n is the viscosity of the fluid, L is the pipe length, π is 3.1416, and r is the radius of the pipe lumen.

Along with its influence on resistance, viscosity plays a central role in the overall stability of flow. Viscosity is a measure of the internal friction that exists within a fluid or gas.[5] It is the resistance offered by a fluid or gas to a nonaccelerating displacement of adjacent particle layers. The dimensions for this resistance are force $\times$ time per unit area of contact. The cgs (centimeter gram second) viscosity unit is the *poise,* and for most biological fluids, the *centipoise.*

The relationship between contributors to flow resistance and flow itself can be illustrated by combining the equation for resistance and Poiseuille's equation:

$$Q = P\,\pi\,r^4/8nL \tag{4.10}$$

Flow (Q) and pressure (P) still vary directly, but the influence of other factors becomes quite clear. For example, flow varies with the fourth power of the radius, which explains why controlling vessel diameter controls the amount of blood traveling through it. Vessel diameter influences not only the flow resistance, but also the volume of a vascular compartment as well. Physiologically, regulation of arterial blood flow to tissues occurs through arteriolar constriction and dilation, in which small changes in vessel radius can enhance or hinder blood flow.

How fast can we push a fluid through a pipe and still have stable flow? The expanded volume-flow equation above shows no limit; nevertheless, a practical limit does exist.

Flow Stability

The obvious way of looking at the question of flow stability is to increase the driving pressure in a model system until flow becomes unstable. Without a view of the fluid, the first evidence of something unusual happening is a change in the pressure-flow relationship. Figure 4-8 shows the graph of pressure (P) and volume flow (V). As the volume flow increases, it suddenly fails to respond to any further increases in driving pressure. A way of understanding what is happening is to follow the fluid streamlines. Normally, the streamlines are smooth and continuous, indicating a stable flow pattern. But in this instance, the streamlines are not smooth, but disturbed and discontinuous.

In the late 1800s, Osborne Reynolds (1842–1912) investigated this problem using large fluid-pipe models.[5] He not only looked at the pressure-flow relationship, but also other parameters such as fluid viscosity and the radius of the lumen. His goal was to determine their influence on the stability of flow through a pipe.

Reynolds found that when a flow pattern became unstable, the normally continuous streamlines broke up, forming small local circular currents called eddy currents and vortices. At this transition between stable and disturbed flow, delivering more energy to the system by increasing pressure did not increase the volume flow; instead, the amount of disturbance increased. The additional energy put into the system by increasing pressure was clearly going only into the eddy current formation.

Reynolds derived a dimensionless number that predicted when a fluid became unstable.[5] The equation for that number contains the major contributors to flow stability:

$$Re = vpr/n \qquad (4.11)$$

where Re is the dimensionless Reynolds number, v is the mean velocity across the pipe, p is the fluid density, r is the lumen radius, and n is the fluid viscosity. If the Reynolds number exceeded 1,000 for a flowing fluid when using the mean velocity within the pipe, or 2,000 when using the maximum velocity in the pipe, the flow became unstable.

One way of using the Reynolds equation is to insert the critical Reynolds number and calculate the critical velocities for a particular flow situation. For example, suppose we wanted to know when blood flow might become unstable and produce a noise or bruit from a vessel, such as the aorta. The critical velocity (V_c) equation is

$$V_c = n(Re)/pr \qquad (4.12)$$

Using 0.04 poise for blood viscosity, 1,000 for Re, 1.0 g/cm³ for blood density, and a 1-cm aortic radius gives

$$V_c = 0.04 \times 1,000 / 1.0 \times 1.0$$

which is about 40 cm/s, a velocity easily possible during early systole.

In general, the Reynolds equation applies to straight, rigid pipes. Nevertheless, it does give the clinician some elementary insight into the physics of flow. Narrowings or dilations in vessels that come from anatomy or disease can cause flow instabilities. Indeed, such flow instabilities, detected with Doppler ultrasound, are the sensitive indicators of flow-disrupting disease. The flexibility of blood vessels coupled with the specific fluid nature of blood (particulates in a moving fluid) can cause some unexpected results. Understanding the basic principles and causes of these unusual results can help the clinician sort out true disease from variations in normal physiology.

The physical forms of a flow disturbance are eddy currents and vortices. Smooth, continuous streamlines appear with laminar flow, which represents the smooth movement of layers or laminations of fluid particles over one another. Eddy currents are circular, backward (relative to the bulk flow) movements of the fluid, and their formation breaks up streamlines (Fig. 4-9A). These disturbances travel downstream, moving along with the bulk flow. Eventually, the movement expends the energy that went into their formation and the currents disappear.

Vortices, in contrast, are a little more complex, taking on a closed form with a stabilizing internal movement. A vortex is like a smoke ring. It has a radial rotation within the body of the ring (Fig. 4-9B). A vortex can travel some distance in a fluid and keep its shape because the internal motion gives the vortex stability. Just like the eddy current, a vortex will eventually expend its energy and disappear.

Eddies and vortices are not just abstract concepts, useful only to the mechanical engineer. They are phenomena that occur in the vascular system of man. In the internal

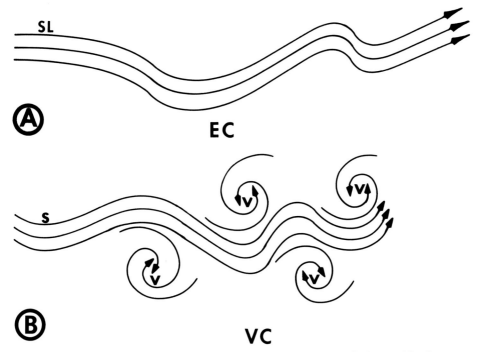

Figure 4-9   Unstable fluid motion. **A**, As fluid motion becomes increasingly unstable, the stream lines (*SL*) begin to waver, forming eddy currents (*EC*). **B**, Putting more energy into the fluid transforms the eddy currents into vortices (*VC*), where each vortex (*v*) becomes a self-contained packet of energy. The vortices come from the fluid turbulence that breaks up the streamlines (*S*).

carotid artery bulb, for example, eddies occur normally and are absent in disease as the bulb partially fills with atheromatous material. Vortices in flow arise as arteries become aneurysmal, and this flow pattern is one of the early markers of arterial dilation. Recent advances in ultrasound imaging that are discussed in later chapters have allowed the clinician to connect these elements of flow physiology with disease.

Expanding the Volume Flow Model

If a long pipe has a complex shape with a variety of narrowings, each narrowing with a different geometry, a good analytical question to ask is: What limits the volume flow through the pipe? Certainly pressure will be one limit. Changing the driving pressure into the pipe changes the flow through that pipe. In a system with rigid walls, the fluid volume flow is constant along the pipe, which means that the section with the highest resistance sets the volume flow rate. This is similar to the electronic analogy that current is constant through a series circuit. And if the volume flow is constant through a pipe, then any narrowing must increase the fluid velocity through that narrowing.

This connection between a lumen narrowing and fluid velocity is easy to see through the conservation of mass. Let's start with a pipe that has two different diameters and pistons at both ends, with one piston larger than the other (Fig. 4-10). The volume displaced by piston 1 is the area A_1 times the piston displacement d_1. When piston 2 moves, it displaces this same volume, which is A_2 times the displacement d_2.

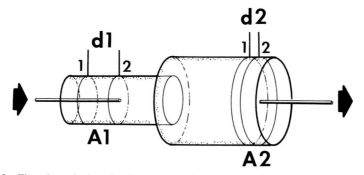

Figure 4-10   Flow through changing lumen sizes. Pushing in the left piston with area *A1* over distance *d1* pushes out the second piston with area *A2* over a distance *d2*. The volume displaced at both pistons is the same. As a result, distance *d2* will be less than *d1*.

The volume flow rate, which we derived earlier is

$$A_1 v_1 = A_2 v_2 \tag{4.13}$$

where v_1 and v_2 are the respective velocities. Putting the areas on one side and the velocities on the other gives

$$A_1/A_2 = v_2/v_1 \tag{4.14}$$

This simple equation says that reducing the cross-sectional area of a pipe (A_2 is larger than A_1) will increase the velocity of the fluid through the narrowing from v_2 to v_1. The actual velocity increase is proportional to the ratio of the area change. From this relationship comes two rules: first, moving from a large lumen to a small lumen increases the fluid velocity; and second, moving from a small lumen to a large lumen decreases the fluid velocity.

Because flow resistance is proportional to the fourth power of the lumen radius, it is instructive to calculate just how flow changes with lumen size. Velocity, we already know, depends on the area of the narrowing. Poiseuille's equation (Eq. 4.8) would indicate that decreasing volume flow to 50% of its original value requires the resistance to double. Application of the resistance equation (Eq. 4.9) would suggest that reducing the radius by 16% reduces the cross-sectional area by nearly 30%, increasing resistance by a factor of two.

In reality, the vascular system is not passive but responds to reduced flow into key organs by increasing the systemic blood pressure.[6] For example, decreased flow and pressure to a baroreceptor in the carotid body will cause the systemic blood pressure to increase. For vascular beds such as the brain and kidney, the systemic blood pressure will increase in response to reduced blood volumes reaching what appear to be "volume receptors."[6] Although the body depends upon the volume of blood reaching the tissues per unit time, it really has no major "volume sensors." Instead, the body senses most of the vascular dynamics through baroreceptors that respond to pressure.[6] The connection between blood pressure and vascular narrowing is that a flow-reducing stenosis reduces downstream pressure. As a result, a flow-decreasing lesion in a major vascular bed often causes the systemic blood pressure to rise as the vascular control system responds to a sensed flow reduction. Thus, hypertension results from renal artery stenosis when a flow-reducing lesion in the renal artery decreases the pressure sensed by the juxtaglomerular apparatus in the renal circulation. This pressure sensitive tissue then releases renin, which ultimately raises blood pressure via the action of angiotensin and aldosterone.

Another View of Flow: Velocity

Up to now, we have viewed flow as a volume transport phenomenon without regard to velocity, other than the average velocity used to calculate volume flow. Real fluids have both mass and friction between the fluid particles. The friction within a fluid eliminates spatially uniform flow velocities in pipes and conduits. This influence of velocity on volume flow is evident from the basic continuity equation

$$Q = V_{avg} A \tag{4.15}$$

where Q is the volume flow rate, V_{avg} is the average spatial velocity, and A is the cross-sectional area. To determine volume flow, we need to understand flow velocity. In turn, velocity yields more than just volume information; it provides an intimate view of the character of flow, a character quickly changed by the presence of disease. Ultimately, the particle velocity distribution in a flow pattern will show whether the fluid movement is stable or unstable. If it is unstable, the pattern shows whether the flow is simply disturbed or very turbulent. At the center of events leading either to stable or unstable flow is fluid viscosity.

Fluid Viscosity   The attraction among particles of a fluid influences its ability to handle shear forces, tangential forces that act parallel to a surface or plane within a fluid. Figure 4-11 shows the appearance of shear forces. Increasing the strength of bonding or viscosity forces in a fluid effectively increases the internal resistance of that fluid. Qualitative evidence of the particle-binding forces appears by observing how a liquid pours from one container to another. For example, as viscosity increases, the fluid becomes thicker and increasingly slow to pour.

A way of quantifying these viscous forces is to measure the force required to move two plates separated by a small thickness of fluid.[7] This measurement requires putting the fluid between two large cylinders and rotating one cylinder around the other. This geometry, shown in Figure 4-12, permits a measurement of how much energy it takes to overcome the viscous forces.

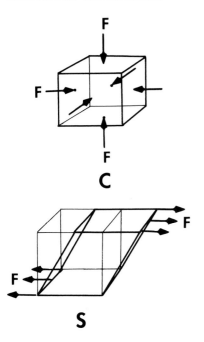

Figure 4-11   Compression and shear forces. Compressional forces (*C*) in fluids press on the fluid from all directions. All the forces (*F*) point toward a single point. In contrast, shear (*S*) forces exert a torque around a single point, with the force vectors (*F*) in opposite directions. Fluids can support compressional forces but not shear forces.

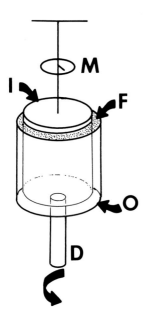

Figure 4-12   Measurement of fluid viscosity. Measuring fluid viscosity or internal resistance begins by driving (*D*) an outside container (*O*) that surrounds an inside cylinder (*I*). The fluid (*F*) sits between the two surfaces. As the external motion couples to the inner surface through the fluid, a torque appears on the inner cylinder that registers on a meter (*M*). The greater the viscosity, the greater the torque.

Issac Newton (1643–1727) first proposed the model for fluid motion in which laminations or layers of fluid particles move against one another.[6] Figure 4-13 shows the geometry of this concept. When fluids move this way, we call the flow laminar, and fluids that behave this way are called Newtonian fluids.

Movement of a viscous fluid through a pipe will set up shear forces within that fluid. A shear force gradient is set up by a stationary layer of liquid at the wall of the pipe. The fastest moving segment of the fluid is in the center of the lumen.

Stable Flow in a Pipe   A steady driving pressure initiates movement of a viscous fluid through a pipe. Without a change in pressure down the pipe, the fluid will not move. If the fluid velocity produces a Reynolds number below the critical value, fluid movement is stable, and flow is laminar. At the walls of the pipe, the fluid forms a stationary boundary layer with zero velocity. The center of the lumen, in contrast, is the site of the maximum velocity.

In general, the spatial velocity distribution, extending from a zero-velocity layer at the wall to the highest velocity region in the center, takes on a specific shape. This shape is a parabola in two dimensions and a paraboloid in three dimensions (Fig. 4-13), giving this form of flow its name: parabolic. The average velocity for a three-dimensional paraboloid is half the maximum velocity. As with the simpler flow patterns discussed earlier, parabolic fluid flow is governed by Poiseuille's equation (Eq. 4.8) and the basic volume flow equation (Eqs. 4.3 and 4.15).

Viscous forces within a fluid represent a source of energy loss always converting some of the work done on the fluid by outside forces into heat.[8] This heat loss is similar to the frictional energy losses associated with moving solid bodies over one another. The stationary fluid interface between a pipe wall and liquid is called the boundary layer. It must theoretically and practically satisfy the boundary conditions of having the same velocity as the walls of the pipe, which is zero. Under stable conditions, the boundary layer remains in contact with the wall. During some instabilities, however, the fluid boundary layer can leave the wall and reattach downstream, forming a flow pattern called a separation.

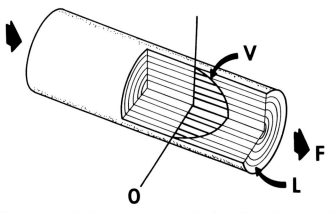

Figure 4-13 Laminar parabolic flow pattern. In a straight pipe with steady state conditions, the flow (*F*) velocity profile takes the shape of a parabola (*V*), with a boundary layer right at the pipe-fluid interface (*0 line*). Within the fluid, flow occurs as small layers or lamellae (*L*) of material move over one another.

Unstable Flow   As shown in Figure 4-8, increasing the driving pressure to a pipe will steadily increase the volume flow. Increasing the driving pressure further, however, produces a lower rate of flow increase, or no increase in volume flow at all. This forms the transition from a stable to an unstable flow pattern.

   Within the fluid, instabilities begin to deform the streamlines. As the average velocity increases, the instabilities take up greater amounts of energy, eventually breaking down the continuity of surrounding streamlines, mixing the fluid moving in adjacent streamlines. The instabilities begin to generate eddy currents and vortices that travel down the pipe with the moving fluid. This divides the flow into two components, the average velocity that produces the bulk volume flow down the pipe and the local flow of eddy currents and vortices. These currents can have both forward and reverse velocity components (Fig. 4-14). In this situation, the shape of the average velocity across the pipe becomes blunt. At the same time, variations in velocity at each point on the average velocity wave front can be quite large.[5]

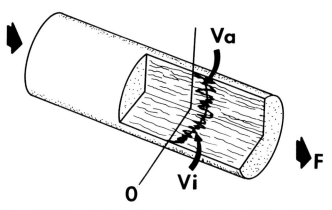

Figure 4-14 Flow with in-line turbulence. Flow can be unstable and still maintain bulk flow characteristics. The velocity profile includes a boundary layer at the wall (*0 line*) and a blunt-appearing average velocity (*Va*). The small regional flow velocities (*Vi*), however, are very irregular. The irregularities represent disrupted streamlines that may be continuous over only small portions of the flow pattern.

Thus, increasing the driving pressure does not increase the amount of volume flow within such a system. Instead, the disturbances increase, with all the additional energy being converted into disturbed motion. The viscous forces within the fluid continue to work, and much of this additional energy becomes heat.

Just as unstable flow can break the organization of streamlines, it can also destroy the continuity of the fluid-wall contact. When this happens, the boundary layer completely separates from the wall, becoming a free fluid surface. The result is a flow separation. At the separation site, the streamline becomes mathematically discontinuous as it suddenly heads off in a new direction, no longer following the walls of the pipe or container.[5] An everyday example is pouring a fluid from a container. As a fluid separates from the container wall, or as water flows out the free end of a pipe, separations are easy to see. Within an enclosed fluid system, a separation can look like a jet flowing into a much slower fluid volume. These phenomena are observed in patients with arteriovenous fistulas created for hemodialysis. In this situation, the laminar, arterial, high-pressure flow enters a low-pressure venous conduit. The result is a complete loss of streamlines, with boundary layer separation and eddy current formations at the connection between artery and vein. Energy also dissipates from the vessels as a mechanical vibration of the adjacent tissue. Farther downstream from the anastamosis, venous flow resumes a laminar pattern with streamlines and a boundary layer. The elements of flow separation appear in Figure 4-15.

Flow separations leave behind regions with very little or no movement.[5] They are areas of flow stagnation. In a pulsatile system, some of these separations will have short periods of reverse flow as the traveling pulse wave sets up local pressure gradients. These spatial pressure differences move the fluid within the separation bubble in a direction opposite to the general fluid motion.

This is precisely the situation that seems to occur in the normal internal carotid artery. Most individuals have a dilated portion of the artery known as the carotid bulb. When blood enters this dilated portion of the artery during systole, a flow separation occurs with a resulting reversed flow in the separation bubble. Farther downstream, the streamlines contact the wall and reestablish the boundary layer. These conditions are shown in Figure 4-16.

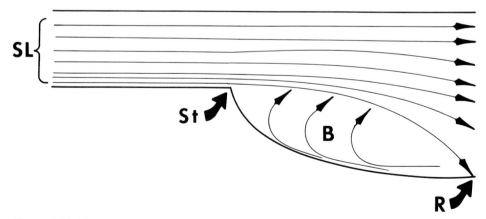

Figure 4-15   Flow separation process. A flow separation occurs when the streamlines (*SL*) near the wall detach (*St*) to form a separation bubble (*B*). It later reattaches to the wall (*R*). This form of separation occurs because the container wall moves away from the streamlines faster than the fluid can respond. Within the separation bubble, flow may be stagnant or reversed in different parts of a pulsatile flow pattern.

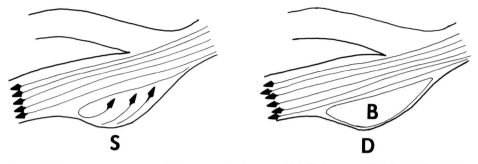

Figure 4-16 Schematic events of flow separation in a carotid bulb. In a carotid bulb, the flow in the separation is reversed during systole (*S*) because of a strong pressure gradient between the separation segment and the fast-moving blood. In diastole (*D*), the slowing blood flow makes the two pressures nearly the same and the separation bubble (*B*) becomes stagnant, with little or no flow.

Flow separations depend heavily on the geometry of the containing pipe. Rapid changes in diameter, bends, and kinks all create situations in which the streamline next to the boundary layer cannot follow the changing geometry. In the vascular system, these are conditions often associated with arterial bifurcations, dilations, and tortuosities. Figure 4-17 displays an example of vascular flow separation (see color section between pp. 116 and 117).

Aid and Comfort from Bernoulli

It is hardly an exaggeration to say that the Bernoulli equation is at the center of hydrodynamics. It will even play a central role in the quantitative applications of Doppler.

As discussed earlier, the streamline traces out particle motion in the fluid. Stable flow means the streamlines are unbroken. This is the primary condition for applying the Bernoulli equation, which follows the changes in energy along the streamline.

Bernoulli's equation makes the primary assumption that the total energy along a streamline is constant. The energy simply changes from one form to another as the conditions surrounding the streamline change. In the equation, pressure appears as a form of potential energy. Although pressure potentiates the other forms of energy, it is not the only reason for fluid movement. Another contributor to total energy is hydrostatic pressure. And a moving fluid with mass also has kinetic energy. These energy segments combine to form the Bernoulli equation

$$P + pv^2/2 + pgh = \text{constant} \tag{4.16}$$

where P is pressure, p is fluid density, v is particle velocity, g is gravitational acceleration, and h is height in the gravitational field. Or in broader terms, P is the potential energy, $pv^2/2$ is the kinetic energy, and pgh is the hydrostatic pressure. Along a streamline, then, we can write the following equation

$$P_1 + pv_1^2/2 + pgh_1 = P_2 + pv_2^2/2 + pgh_2 \tag{4.17}$$

where 1 and 2 are points along the same streamline. This equation says that the sum of energies at point 1 is equal to the sum of energies at point 2. Solving for pressure yields

$$P_1 - P_2 = \tfrac{1}{2} p(v_2^2 - v_1^2) + pg \, (h^2 - h_1) \tag{4.18}$$

which shows the conversion of potential energy (pressure) into kinetic energy and hydrostatic pressure, respectively. Let's look at each of these terms a little more closely.

Pressure acts like potential energy in fluids.[2] It is analogous to voltage in electronics: both can exist without motion. Just as voltage can extend to the end of a wire without an electrical current, pressure can extend to the end of a capped hose without fluid flow. Uncapping the hose permits the fluid to move. Motion means velocity, and in a fluid with mass, imparting motion gives the fluid kinetic energy. In this way, potential energy (pressure) is transformed into kinetic energy. The kinetic energy term is

$$\tfrac{1}{2}\, pv^2 \tag{4.19}$$

where p is the mass density of the fluid and v is the particle velocity along the streamline at any point.

Energy is also available from the external gravitational field in the form of hydrostatic pressure. This term looks like pgh, where p is the mass density of the fluid, g is the gravitational acceleration, and h is the height of the fluid within the gravitational field. Figure 4-18 shows the physical events surrounding the Bernoulli equation.

In the simple Bernoulli equation, the moving fluid shifts energy from one form to another, depending upon the local conditions. At the same time, the *total* energy remains constant. If the flow is horizontal, then the hydrostatic pressure makes no contribution and the equation reduces to

$$P_1 - P_2 = \tfrac{1}{2}\, p\, (v_2^2 - v_1^2) \tag{4.20}$$

which says that the pressure difference between any two points on a streamline is a function of the difference in particle kinetic energy or, in other words, the particle velocities. And because the pressure and the kinetic energy at a point sum to a constant, an *increase* in local velocity will produce a *decrease* in local pressure. This is known as the *Venturi effect*.[7]

If a fluid has no velocity (i.e., is stationary), then it will have no kinetic energy. In this instance, the equation reduces to

$$P + pgh = \text{constant} \tag{4.21}$$

for each point in the system. Furthermore, if the constant is zero, then the equation becomes

$$P = -pgh \tag{4.22}$$

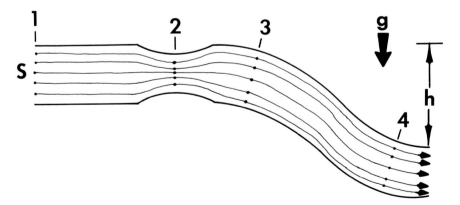

Figure 4-18   Elements in the Bernoulli equation. The streamlines (S) enter the lumen at position *1*. At position *2*, the narrowing causes an increase in velocity and kinetic energy, producing a lower pressure. At position *3*, the kinetic energy and velocity reduce again, and pressure is restored. Moving from position *3* to position *4* creates a hydrostatic head that is a function of the change in height (h) and gravitational acceleration (g). With continuous flow, the sum of all the energy forms is a constant.

which is the equation for hydrostatic pressure we looked at earlier (Eq. 4.1). This equation also explains why a fluid in an open flask does not flow out because of an apparent pressure difference. In fact, the net energy of the fluid is zero everywhere in the flask, and as the Bernoulli equation shows, fluids move down energy gradients, not just pressure gradients. The result is a stable glass of water.

Making the Bernoulli Equation More Real

Two aspects of the simple Bernoulli equation are clear. First, the equation does not handle any energy loss through flow resistance. In addition, it has no inertial terms to handle the energy changes during acceleration and deceleration of the fluid. Modifying the simplified Bernoulli equation for these energy terms makes it more real and, in that way, a better tool for quantitative Doppler applications.

The vascular system is driven by a pulsatile train of heart beats. In each cycle, the blood must start and stop, which means the vascular system expends energy to overcome the inertia of the blood. Basically, inertia means that blood at rest likes to stay at rest, and blood in motion likes to stay in motion. (Newton's first law, simply stated, is that bodies in motion stay in motion, and bodies at rest stay at rest—does that sound familiar?)

Accelerating a fluid with mass takes energy, and this delays the response of the fluid to the driving pressure. The work required to move a particle is equal to the force on the particle times the distance it moves, which in this case, is along a streamline. The total work is the sum of all the little pieces of work along the way. Each little piece of work is added to all the others through an integral which appears as

$$p \int (dV/dt) dl \qquad (4.23)$$

where p is the mass density, V is the particle velocity along the streamline, and dl is a very small line segment along the streamline and a vector quantity (it has magnitude and direction).

Fluid resistance can be as simple as internal viscous forces or as complex as the resistance afforded by a pipe or conduit carrying fluid. Essential to this form of energy loss is movement. This term is directly proportional to the velocity and is expressed as

$$RV$$

where R is the fluid resistance and V is the instantaneous velocity along a streamline.

Combining terms, the modified Bernoulli equation takes the verbal form

Total energy = potential energy + kinetic energy +
work to accelerate + work to overcome fluid resistance.

Mathematically, the equation appears as

$$P + (\tfrac{1}{2})pV^2 + pgh + p \int (dV/dt) dl + RV = \text{constant} \qquad (4.24)$$

The modified Bernoulli equation can be a valuable clinical tool. Cardiologists can estimate the pressure gradient across a stenotic aortic valve by using Doppler to measure the maximum velocity through the valve. Vascular surgeons, using similar Doppler techniques, have accurately estimated the significance of flow-limiting lesions in the extremities. Applying the Bernoulli equation to determine pressure differences by measuring velocity requires that the other terms become insignificant, i.e., too small to contribute. For example, if a stenotic valve becomes small enough and the fluid velocity high enough, the velocity-dependent, resistance term begins to affect results, creating an underestimate of the real pressure gradient.[8]

Time-Dependent Pressure: Pulsatile Flow

The energy that moves blood through the vascular system comes from the heart. Up to now, a steady pressure has been the assumption. Introducing a rhythmic driving force not only changes events within a fluid, but also how we must regard such a fluid system. Within each rhythmic event is fluid acceleration, deceleration, and rest. These represent very "nonsteady" conditions that affect fluid behavior over space and time. In addition, the rhythm of the driving energy allows frequency-dependent mechanisms in fluid flow to take effect.[4] Differences between pulsatile and steady flow are as large as the differences between direct current and alternating current circuits in electronics.

Acceleration represents the start of events. In early acceleration, before significant movement exists, the driving pressure spreads uniformly throughout a fluid. Thus acceleration across the lumen of a pipe is uniform. This uniform delivery of pressure is, of course, Pascal's law. Movement involves velocity dependent terms, however, including inertia and fluid resistance. As a result, the fluid delays its response to the applied pressure because of inertia. Then, as movement occurs, the pressure becomes nonuniform across the lumen. As the nonuniform response increases, the center stream ultimately moves the fastest and the boundary layer at the pipe wall moves the least.

Depending upon the inertia of a fluid, its maximum velocity and the maximum pressure are not temporally together. For example, the movement trails behind the changing pressure throughout the heart cycle, and some of the applied energy goes into this acceleration process.

During the deceleration phase, the distribution of energy is not uniform among streamlines, but the energy is constant along each streamline. As a result, momentum has a greater effect in the higher velocity regions of a fluid flow pattern. Therefore, slowing is not evenly distributed within the fluid as the driving pressure decreases. If a fluid is carrying particles (e.g., blood carrying erythrocytes) deceleration appears more disruptive and disorganized than acceleration, because the early acceleration has none of the pressure differences or velocity differences that appear later in the cycle. These disruptive qualities of deceleration appear in the Doppler signals returning from moving blood. Figure 4-19 summarizes these events common to most pulsatile flow situations.

New Doppler ultrasound technology removes the earlier concepts in this discussion from the theories of fluid flow and places them in the center of clinical medicine. Physicians can now recognize flow patterns that occur over different parts of the cardiac cycle in normal vessels such as carotid arteries. Jets, boundary layer separations, and flow deviations predicted from hydrodynamic principles can all be identified in the healthy human body. Alterations in these normal patterns have been described and are now utilized in diagnosing disease.

Hydrodynamics: A Summary

A pivotal concept to come from this discussion is that fluids move down energy gradients, not just pressure gradients. In addition, the energy of a fluid particle traveling

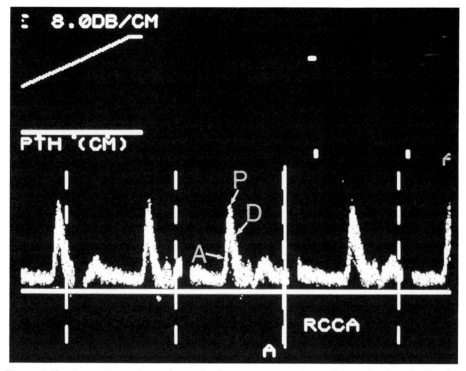

Figure 4-19 Spectral waveform of vascular flow events over the cardiac cycle. Systolic flow in a vessel consists of an acceleration (*A*), a peak velocity (*P*), and a deceleration period (*D*). Flow may or may not exist in diastole. It does in this example of a common carotid artery. In general, flow is more organized in acceleration, producing a narrower range of Doppler frequencies. Deceleration, however, is more disorganized, producing a wider range of Doppler shift frequencies.

along a streamline is constant, and in laminar flow situations, the Bernoulli equation permits a calculation of fluid dynamics.

Because of the streamlines and the conservation of mass, a change in lumen areas will alter the velocity of a fluid. Moving from a large area to a smaller area increases the fluid velocity; moving from a small area to a larger area decreases the fluid velocity.

Laminar flow is stable flow in the sense that the streamlines remain intact. In contrast, unstable flow leads to broken, discontinuous streamlines that finally form into eddy currents and vortices. The stability of a fluid can be reasonably predicted by the Reynolds number, a dimensionless number that depends upon the fluid and velocity conditions that influence flow stability.

As a fluid moves down a pipe, the resistance to flow will depend upon the length of the pipe and the viscosity of the fluid. It will depend the most on the diameter of the pipe, because resistance is a function of the fourth power of the lumen radius. And knowing resistance and the driving pressure, Poiseuille's equation permits a calculation of the volume flow rate.

In general, steady pressure situations are easy to deal with, introducing rather predictable behavior. Pulsatile flow, however, changes both the conditions of the driving pressure as well as the response of the system. Introducing a rhythm to the driving pressure creates time variations between the pressure and the flow response, and involves frequency-dependent characteristics of the fluid and the system.

The Physical Characteristics of Blood

Blood as a Fluid

As a fluid, blood is anything but ideal. Because it carries a variety of particulates that can interact biochemically, blood can take on qualities that never appear in a model consisting of water with small rubber-like particles inside. Whole blood has the following characteristics[9]: a specific gravity of about 1.0595 (1.0964 for erythrocytes); a relative viscosity in vitro of 4.75 centipoise at 18°C (room temperature); and a dynamic viscosity in vivo that ranges from 2.30 to 2.75 centipoise.[18] Blood, of course, is non-rigid, but clotting mechanisms can change the flowing quality of blood very quickly. In general, viscosity can be quite variable in a biological system, whether it is normal or diseased.

Polycythemia rubra vera is a disease process that has a profound effect on blood viscosity and hemodynamics. In this disorder, the patient has a marked increase in the concentration of circulating erythrocytes. This increased cell count significantly increases the viscosity of the blood. Considering the hydrodynamics we have examined up to now, it is possible to predict some complications of this disease. As the viscosity increases, the resistance to flow also increases. In the smaller blood vessels, the increased resistance produces very slow flow. Blood that is slowed or stagnant is increasingly exposed to stimulants that can cause clotting and thrombus formation along the vessel walls. The clots, in turn, produce infarctions in both myocardium and brain.

Blood as a Tissue

Blood makes up about 7% of the total body weight.[9] As a tissue, it comprises a carrying medium called plasma and many formed particles and cells. Cellular components include erythrocytes or red blood cells (RBCs), leukocytes or white blood cells (WBCs), and thrombocytes or platelets, all suspended in a plasma rich in proteins (albumin, immunoglobulins, and carrier proteins).

RBCs make up the largest population of cells, averaging some 5.2 million/mm^3 for men and 4.5 million/mm^3 in women.[9] These cells are discoid, measuring 7 to 10 μm in diameter and about 2 μm thick. RBCs are the major source of backscattering signals for Doppler ultrasound, although not necessarily as individuals; calculations based on ultrasound scattering from blood suggest an effective scattering unit size of 30 to 50 μm.[10] Thus, Doppler signals actually reflect from groups of moving RBCs. Such groups can take the form of long chains called Rouleauxs,[11] which seem to be the source of echo signals often seen in real-time images of larger veins.

Occupying a smaller volume of the vascular system are the WBCs. Even when elevated in number by disease, they remain too few to affect the ultrasonic properties of blood.[13] They do, however, greatly influence the physiological aspects of blood and its role in body immunity. Being particulates, they contribute to the overall fluid qualities of blood as well. WBCs usually number 5,000 to 9,000/mm^3.[9] In disease states such as leukemia, in which the count and size of the WBCs increase, these cells can affect blood flow by increasing blood viscosity. The result can be sludging and thrombosis. The clinician can detect this flow-slowing process with Doppler.

Thrombocytes or platelets are much smaller than RBCs but number about 250,000/mm^3.[9] They contribute to the clotting mechanism of blood, and as such, play a role in the maintenance of vascular integrity. Like WBCs, these particulates are few in number, adding little to either the moving fluid properties of blood or the blood-ultrasound interaction. But as with the other particulates, overactivity of platelets can cause end-organ thrombosis, which can be clinically relevant. And thrombosis is detectable with Doppler ultrasound.

Blood, as a tissue and as a fluid, moves through a set of flexible pipes that respond to hormonal and neural influences as well as disease.

The Vascular System

Two major characteristics affect our view of the vascular system with Doppler: first, the energy travels through the system in pulses; and second, the fluid conduits are flexible, responding actively and passively to internal and external pressures and activities. The pulsatile delivery of pressure provides a look at the hydraulic response of the vascular system with each beat. Pulsatile flow introduces frequency-dependent parameters as the shape of a pulse introduces a wide range of frequencies into the vessels. The flexibility of the vessels will influence the transmission of pulse pressure and the resistance the heart experiences with each beat.

Using Doppler ultrasound, physicians can clinically evaluate the heart as a pump. Two-dimensional, real-time ultrasound and M-mode ultrasound will give us a view of the heart's mechanics, including muscle contraction, valve opening and closing, and integrity.[13] Doppler ultrasound, on the other hand, will examine the moving blood through this pump (cardiac output and stroke volume), giving information on the impediments to flow (pressure gradients and valve areas) and completeness of flow (regurgitation).[8]

Pumping blood into a system of flexible pipes produces a passive volume expansion within a vascular network. This stores some of the driving energy in the elastic elements of the vascular bed, and some of this energy is recovered between pulses.[3] As the vessels contract, blood flows through the vascular bed at a smoother, steadier rate. This model of blood flow into a flexible vascular system is called the Windkessel model. We can witness this effect when the heart ejection expands the aorta, storing energy in the vessel's elastic components. Flow in the more distal portions of the aorta continues throughout the heart cycle, first from cardiac ejection, then from the collapsing vascular walls. The pulse generated by cardiac and aortic contraction travels as a wave, moving along at 5 to 10 m/s.[3]

Fluid Behavior of the Blood

Within the vascular compartment, the blood conforms to all the fluid mechanics we have examined up to now. As a fluid velocity difference forms within the vascular compartment, the Venturi effect (predicted by the Bernoulli equation) makes the pressure within the higher velocity region less than that in the slow region. The RBCs respond to this pressure gradient and migrate toward the higher velocity region.[14] Because the RBCs are already well packed, this effect is not major; but in general, the hematocrit is higher in the center of a vessel than along its edges.[14]

In vessels with diameters greater than 1 mm, blood generally behaves like an ideal Newtonian fluid.[14] At vessel diameters less than 1 mm, however, the particulates begins to influence flow behavior, and blood can look decidedly non-Newtonian.[14] Regardless of vessel diameter, blood conforms to Newton's first law that things tend to move in straight lines. As a consequence, in curving vessels and compartments, peak velocities move away from the central axis.

Blood flow can become unstable in a number of normal situations as well as in the presence of disease. The critical Reynolds number for blood in a straight pipe, for example, is about 1,000, but it can be as low as 150 for small vessels.[15] Flow separations are not uncommon at areas of rapid expansion where the streamlines can not follow the geometry of the vessel wall. Semistagnation areas can form under these circumstances. As a result, some regions experience movement only during a portion of the heart cycle while flow is continuous in other areas of the very same vessel segment. Flow reversals can occur in these stagnation regions when surrounding blood flow has a lower pressure than the slower or stationary blood (Fig. 4-16). These flow mechanics become clinically valuable when trying to diagnose disease in the carotid arteries. The off-center streamlines and flow separations represent normal flow characteristics. In contrast, higher velocities near the center of the vessel with no flow separation can often show atherosclerotic deposition and disease.

Instabilities in blood flow can also occur at wall irregularities that extend into the flow boundary layer. At these sites, the disturbed and broken streamlines form eddy currents and vortices that travel down the vessel.

Behavior at a Stenosis

Proximal to a stenosis, blood behaves like a Newtonian fluid, forming a velocity gradient across the vessel lumen as it moves. Entering the stenosis, however, requires that the flow velocity increase because of a decreasing cross-sectional area. Within the stenosis, flow can be fast and still be stable; in other words, the blood maintains its streamlines and organization. Moving back into the larger opening, however, produces an unstable flow pattern. At the outflow orifice of the stenosis is usually a flow separation, producing a stagnant region around the narrowing (Fig. 4-20). In the center, the high-velocity jet flows into the larger opening, creating flow reversals, eddy currents, and vortices. As flow continues down the vascular compartment, the energy given over to the flow turbulence dissipates, and stability returns to the flowing blood.

Blood Behavior in Larger Vessels

As stated earlier, the blood within vessels significantly larger than 1 mm most often behaves like a Newtonian fluid. For the larger vessels such as the aorta and pulmonary artery, ventricular ejection produces a blunt velocity flow pattern. The blunt pattern remains intact some distance along these vessels.[16] This behavior is instrumental in estimating cardiac output and stroke volume using Doppler ultrasound in the ascending aorta. The blunt profile is, of course, a result of acceleration and flow entry into the vessels. Acceleration comes from the contracting heart, and the flow entry mechanism occurs as blood moves from the larger cross-sectional area of the ventricle into the smaller area of the aorta.

As the pulse travels down the smaller vessels into the peripheral circulation, the pulse waves reflect from changes in hydraulic impedance. These reflections are a lot like ultrasonic reflections from acoustic impedance changes. A vascular bifurcation represents a change in hydraulic impedance, for example, and a portion of the incident energy reflects upstream from the bifurcation. The reflection is in phase with the inci-

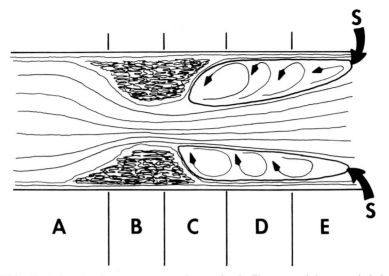

Figure 4-20 Typical regional events at a vessel stenosis. **A,** Flow toward the stenosis is laminar, filling the residual lumen. **B,** The flow accelerates into the stenosis, increasing momentum and kinetic energy. **C,** Flow leaves the narrowing as a high-velocity jet with a high-velocity gradient toward the jet boundaries. The high velocity sets up the proximal portion of the separation bubble (*S*). **D,** Velocity-dependent pressure gradients set up reverse flow within the separation bubbles (*curved arrows*). **E,** As the flow slows, the streamlines fill out the residual lumen again, and stable flow resumes.

dent pressure wave and reinforces it. As a result, the peak pulse pressure amplitude becomes larger as it enters vessels with downward changing hydraulic impedance.

Behavior in the Heart

Within the heart, flow through the valves usually occurs with very small pressure differences from one side to the other.[17] The inflow valves normally impose little impedance to forward flow over the valve, but block retrograde flow when the heart contracts and the valve cusps close. They function like mechanical diodes, and like the electronic version, permit easy flow in one direction and block flow in the other. As the valves narrow with disease, however, it takes more energy to push the blood across them, and moving blood through the heart becomes more difficult. As the stenosis increases, transvalve pressure difference increases.

Filling the atria is largely a passive process, where the kinetic energy of the blood carries flow forward from the vena cavas and pulmonary veins into the atria. Even filling the ventricles is largely passive, with 60% to 80% of the total filling normally occurring during the first (passive) filling phase of the ventricle.[8] Atrial contraction completes the filling, which is the active filling segment of the cardiac cycle.

Ventricular filling seems to create a very large vortex. This filling pattern is quite visible in models of the heart. The vortex pattern becomes apparent as fluid movement into a ventricular shaped cavity is carefully traced out.[19] M-mode and two-dimensional echocardiography show motion patterns of both the mitral and tricuspid valve leaflets that suggest the same sort of filling.[20] Recent advances in Doppler color flow mapping that illustrate the flow patterns within the ventricle further substantiate this filling pattern.[21]

On the outflow side of the cycle, the energy of ventricular contraction converts to pressure because blood is effectively incompressible. When intraventricular pressure exceeds the aortic pressure on the left side and the pulmonary pressure on the right, the ventricles eject blood into the ascending portions of these two arteries. This ejection process accelerates the blood into the great vessels, producing a blunt flow pattern.

Blood Characteristics: A Summary

This discussion has introduced the complexity of pressure and flow patterns in the cardiovascular system. The early clinical use of Doppler ultrasound was hampered by the oversimplified notion of blood as a perfect Newtonian fluid in all clinical circumstances. Even the idea of vessels as semirigid, linear pipes was a comfortable but untrue concept. Clearly, the early, simple models of blood flow are not reliable ways of converting Doppler shift frequencies into reliable blood flow velocities. As advanced imaging systems using color and angiodynography illustrate, our simple assumptions about blood flow are untrustworthy.

In the old model, we thought of a massless blood that moved through inflexible pipes. In reality, blood has mass, momentum, and kinetic energy when in motion, and vessels hardly ever follow straight lines in the body. As a result, blood flow does not always fill a vascular compartment throughout the cardiac cycle. For example, the portions of flow with the greatest kinetic energy continue to move even as the driving energy decreases in diastole. The velocity profiles are not simple parabolas either, but form rather complex geometries. These shapes seldom have the maximum velocities occupying the center of the vessel. And all too often, these high-velocity streamlines are not parallel with the vessel walls.

Despite these complexities, some simplifications can evolve into equations that permit the calculation of pressure gradients, valve areas, and volume flows through the heart and vessels. In general, the understanding that comes from this chapter will pave the way for comprehending the events that are depicted in the color images of flow and the wave forms of a Doppler spectrum.

References

1. Meyer, RE. *Introduction to Mathematical Fluid Dynamics.* New York: Dover Publications, 1971.
2. Halliday, D, and Resnick, R. *Physics for Students of Science and Engineering.* New York: John Wiley and Sons, 1960, pp 357, 362, 378, 424.
3. Milnor, WR. Principles of hemodynamics. *In* Mountcastle, VB (ed): *Medical Physiology,* ed 12. St Louis: The C.V. Mosby, 1968, pp 101–117.
4. Bergel, DH. Blood flow dynamics. *In* Perronneau, P and Diebold, B (eds): *Cardiovascular Applications of Doppler Echography.* Publication 111. Paris: Institut National de la Sante et de la Recherche Medicale, 1982, pp 65–80.
5. Rouse, H. *Elementary Mechanics of Fluids.* New York: Dover, 1946, pp 10, 24, 150, 172, 179.
6. Jensen, D. *The Principles of Physiology.* New York: Appleton-Century-Crofts, 1976, pp 627, 672, 677.
7. Sears, FW, and Zemansky, MW. *College Physics,* ed 3. Reading, MA: Addison-Wesley, 1960, pp 171, 174.
8. Hatle, L, and Angelsen, B. *Doppler Ultrasound in Cardiology.* Philadelphia: Lea & Febiger, 1982, pp 24, 77, Chapter 5.

9. Diem, K, and Lentner, C (eds). *Documenta Geigy Scientific Tables,* ed 7. Basle: Ciba-Geigy, 1970, pp 554, 557.

10. Hanss, M, and Boynard, M. Ultrasound backscattering from blood: Hematocrit and erythrocyte aggregation dependence. *In* Linzer, M (ed): *Ultrasonic Tissue Characterization II,* National Bureau of Standards Special Publication 525. Washington, DC: US Government Printing Office, 1979, pp 165–169.

11. Bloom, W, and Fawcett, DW. *A Textbook of Histology,* ed 9. Philadelphia: WB Saunders, 1968, p 113.

12. Atkinson, P, and Woodcock, JP. *Doppler Ultrasound and Its Use in Clinical Measurement.* New York: Academic Press. 1982, p 5.

13. Roelendt, J. Cardiac cross-sectional anatomy and examination techniques. *Practical Echocardiology.* Forest Grove, OR: Research Studies Press, 1977, Chapter 2.

14. Ganong, WF. *Review of Medical Physiology,* ed 4. Los Altos, CA: Lange Medical Publications, 1969, pp 462–463.

15. Burton, AC. *Physiology and Biophysics of the Circulation.* Chicago: Year Book Medical, 1965, p 134.

16. Merillon, JP, Curien, ND, Touche, T, et al. Vitesse Du Sang Et Profils De Velocité Dans La Crosse Aortique. *In* Peronneau, P and Diebold, B (eds): *Cardiovascular Applications of Doppler Echography,* publication 111. Paris: Institut National de la Sante et de la Recherche Medicale, 1982, pp 295–312.

17. Milnor, WR. The heart as a pump. *In* Mountcastle, VB (ed): *Medical Physiology,* ed 12. St. Louis: CV Mosby, 1968, pp 79–100.

18. Robinson, TF, Factor, SM, and Sonnenblick, EH. The heart as a suction pump. *Sci Am* 254(6):84–91, 1986.

19. Bellhouse, B, and Williams, W. From left atrium to left ventricle. *In* Peronneau, P and Diebold, B (eds): *Cardiovascular Applications of Doppler Echography,* publication 111. Paris: Institut National de la Sante et de la Recherche Medicale, 1982, pp 411–426.

20. Lutas, EM, Devereux, RB, Borer, JS, et al. Echocardiographic evaluation of mitral stenosis: A critical appraisal of its clinical value in detection of severe stenosis and of valvular calcification. *J Cardiovasc Ultrasonography* 2:131–139, 1983

21. Omoto, R (ed). *Color Atlas of Real-Time Two-Dimensional Doppler Echocardiography.* Tokyo: Shidan-To-Chiryo, 1984, p 48.

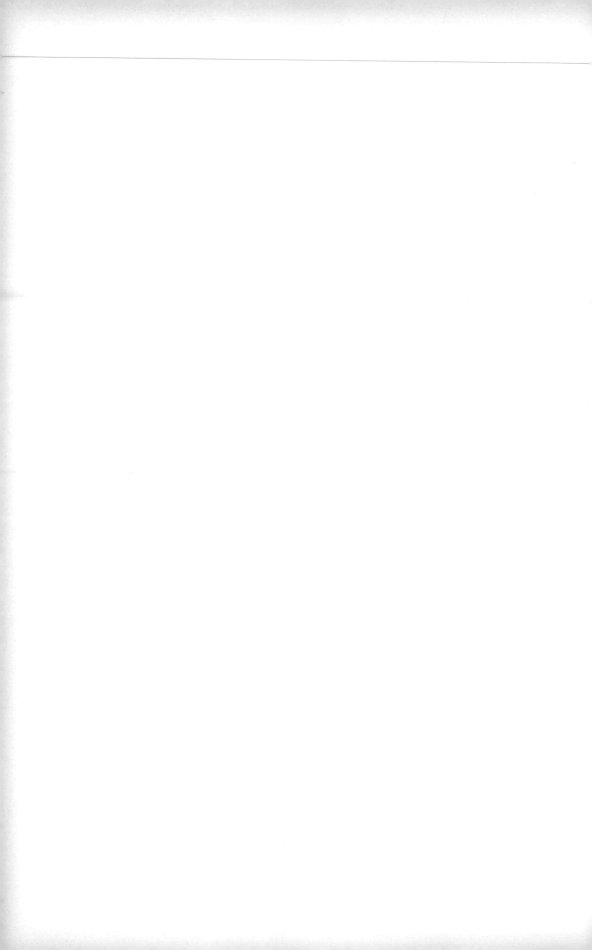

5

The Doppler Equation as a Tool

At the center of Doppler applications of ultrasound is the Doppler equation. In the end, this equation will not only explain how the Doppler effect works, but also outline strategies for solving some scanning problems. It will even lay out the signal processing needs.

This requirement for an equation contrasts with other applications of ultrasound. They do not use an equation as one of the scanning tools, although equations may be part of understanding what is happening. Doppler ultrasound includes too many variables for easy visualization. An equation, on the other hand, is an efficient form of shorthand that can keep a complex relationship in a single, tight, concise expression.

Using the Doppler equation as a tool requires that we understand its roots and what the variables in the equation mean. Deriving this meaning usually involves mathematically building the equation. We could develop the Doppler equation rigorously, but mathematics is not a second language for most of us. A better alternative is to bring the parts of the equation together conceptually, stepping through a series of smaller relationships that ultimately combine to build the final expression. Ultimately, the Doppler equation should not be just a set of letters and numbers. It should express a set of relationships that will turn the equation into an effective tool for thinking about and using Doppler ultrasound.

Origins of the Equation

In 1846, Christian Johann Doppler published his solution to one of the central physics questions of his day: Why do some stars appear red and others appear blue?[1] Perhaps the stars were moving, and on this assumption, Doppler derived an equation to describe these observations. The equation centered on the supposition that sources of light moving away from an observer would have a color shifted toward red, and sources moving toward an observer would have a color shifted toward blue.

This novel thought had very little acceptance within the scientific community. Doppler received all sorts of criticism from his colleagues for what they perceived to be obviously flawed logic in explaining the color of stars.[1] In 1848, however, a Belgian graduate student named Buys Ballow carried out a series of experiments to test the

Doppler equation.[1] He used musicians with perfect pitch (a natural frequency meter) to measure frequency changes as a result of motion. His experiment was rather simple: a musician on a train played a preselected note, while a stationary musician evaluated its pitch as the train moved by. Ballow concluded that the Doppler effect certainly worked for sound, but at the same time, he doubted that it could also work for light.[1]

Modern astronomy finally verified the Doppler effect in light at the turn of the century. It turned out, however, that the Doppler effect was not large enough to change the color of stars as much as Doppler originally suggested.[2] The color of stars depended more on temperature (blue stars are hotter than red stars) than on motion.[2] The Doppler equation, however, became a tool for observing the motion and distance of stars relative to the earth. The Doppler shift did indeed occur for light from moving stars. Ultimately, the Doppler effect happens with all waves, even stationary waves on graph paper, provided the initial conditions are right.

Initial Conditions

The Doppler effect rests on three assumptions about the propagation of waves through a medium. First, the propagation velocity is constant. Second, it is the same in all directions (the medium is said to be isotropic). Third, a wave is independent of its source once it propagates into a carrying medium. These assumptions also apply to ultrasound propagation in the tissues. In reality, the propagation velocity of ultrasound does vary a little with frequency (dispersion)[3] and does depend upon direction in some tissues (anisotropy).[4]

With the above conditions being true, a stationary point source of waves would have a symmetrical set of waves moving outward from it into a surrounding propagating medium. This condition is shown in Figure 5-1. The distance between any two successive identical points in the waves is defined by the wavelength-frequency equation

$$c = \lambda f \tag{5.1}$$

where c is the propagation velocity, λ is the wavelength, and f is the wave frequency. As the frequency of a wave increases, the wavelength decreases in a manner that keeps the product of the two a constant. As a consequence, anything that would change the wavelength of a wave would also change its frequency, provided the propagation velocity is constant.

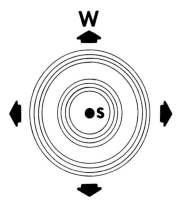

Figure 5-1 Symmetrical wave propagation. Assuming 1) a constant wave velocity, 2) isotropic propagation, and 3) propagating waves that are independent of their source, the waves (W) from a point source (s) will propagate outward, symmetrical to the source.

Central to this model is the independence of the propagating wave and the point source once the wave enters the medium. A source may move or even disappear, but the wave that moved off that source will continue to exist and move through the medium.

With these conditions, two Doppler effects are possible. First, an observer can be moving through a stationary wave field. Second, a stationary observer can be looking at waves from a moving source. For the remainder of this discussion, the moving observer and stationary waves will be the first Doppler effect. In contrast, a stationary observer and moving source will be the second Doppler effect. We look at each of these effects separately, then combine them into a single equation.

First Doppler Effect

The first Doppler effect begins with a stationary source of waves and a moving observer. Initially, if an observer moves along a line connecting the source and observer, the waves seem to increase in frequency because the wave components appear closer together (Fig. 5-2). In other words, the wavelength seems to shrink. If the observer increases speed, the wavelength appears to shrink even more, and the frequency change becomes greater. Slowing down, of course, reduces the effect and the frequency change decreases.

The central condition for this frequency change is motion. If an observer stops, the wave frequency returns to its natural (stationary) value. Thus, for a frequency change to occur, relative motion must exist between the source and the observer.

When the observer moves along the connecting line but away from the wave source, the observed frequency shifts downward, below the stationary value. And just as before, slowing the observer decreases the change in frequency. But now, *increasing*

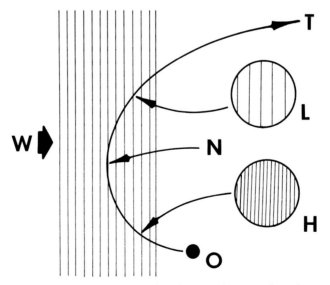

Figure 5-2   The first Doppler effect. As a moving observer (*O*) passes through a set of waves (*W*), the observer sees different wave frequencies as a function of the travel direction. Moving toward the wave source decreases the apparent wavelength (*H*), making the frequency appear higher. Moving away increases the apparent wavelength (*L*), making the frequency appear lower. When parallel to the wave fronts (perpendicular to the wave propagation direction), the observer sees no change (*N*) in wave frequency.

the speed of the observer *decreases* the apparent frequency even more. This is really a consequence of our mathematics. The observed frequency decreases toward a zero value. Thus, speeding up the observer increases the frequency change, but the change decreases the observed frequency toward zero. Slowing down moves the observed frequency back toward the stationary value.

These observations become even more complex if our moving observer does not change speed but simply the direction of motion relative to the source (Fig. 5-2). Swerving within a field of waves also changes the apparent frequency. The frequency is highest when the observer moves along the connecting line but steadily decreases as the direction of the motion deviates more and more away from the line. When the direction of motion is 90° to the line, the observed frequency and the stationary frequency become the same.

Based on these observations, a moving observer could draw the following conclusions about the relationship between frequency changes and observer motion:

1. A change in observed frequency depends upon observer motion and changes directly with observer speed.
2. The frequency change also depends upon the direction the observer is moving. The change reaches a peak value when the source and observer move directly toward one another, and goes to zero when motion is 90° to the connecting line between the two.

It is clear that the largest frequency changes occur when the observer is moving directly away from or toward the wave source. When the motion is more oblique, only part of the observer motion brings the observer and source toward or away from each other. And when the observer motion is perpendicular to the connecting line, movement toward or away from each other no longer exists, i.e., no part of that motion changes the length of the line connecting the two bodies. Any motion that brings the source and observer closer together or farther apart is called the closing velocity.

If we treat the observer motion as a velocity vector with both magnitude and direction, the closing velocity takes on a mathematical form. That portion of a velocity vector produced by projecting the vector along the connecting line between source and observer is the closing velocity (also called a vector component) (Fig. 5-3). And following these vector rules, motion perpendicular to the connecting line can have no vector component projected onto the connecting line. With no closing velocity, the shift in frequency goes to zero.

Although the first Doppler effect contributes to the total Doppler effect in echo-ranging ultrasound, it does not provide a good picture of physical events. The second Doppler effect is a better choice.

The Second Doppler Effect

A closing velocity can result from three conditions. First, the observer could be moving and the wave source stationary. Second, the observer could be stationary and the wave source moving. And third, they both could be moving. Depending upon how we reference the motion, two objects moving toward one another can be viewed as if one were stationary and the other moving relative to it. We can choose either one as our reference point. In this case, we choose the source to be moving and the observer to be stationary.

As the wave source moves, the generated waves become spatially distorted (Fig.

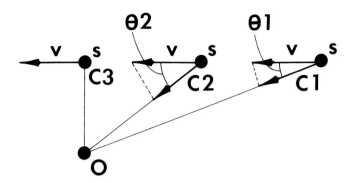

Figure 5-3 Rules governing closing velocity. The closing velocity of a moving source (*s*) is the projection of the source velocity onto the line connecting the source and the observer (*O*). As the angle increases ($\theta 1$, $\theta 2$) toward 90° the closing velocity becomes smaller (*C1, C2, C3*).

5-4). In the direction of motion, they compress; in the other direction, they pull apart. And between these two extremes, the wave length changes steadily, except at 90° to the direction of motion. Here the wave frequency is unchanged. How could this distortion occur? The answer lies in the initial assumptions we made about the behavior of waves in an isotropic medium.

When the source was stationary (Fig. 5-1), it produced a set of concentric waves, symmetrical to itself. The symmetry came from the uniform propagation velocity of the waves. In motion, the source continues to produce waves, but they are no longer concentric to the same point. Instead, each wave is concentric to the point in space where the source was located when the wave left the source and entered the carrying medium. And once the wave entered the medium, it was constrained to move at a uniform velocity, independent of source motion. The result is a moving source that distorts its emitted wave field as shown in Fig. 5-4.

Examination of this distorted field shows that although the frequency does not go to zero anywhere, the change in frequency does. Again, we observe a connection be-

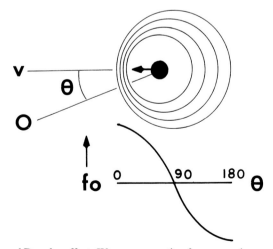

Figure 5-4 The second Doppler effect. Waves propagating from a moving source are distorted spatially. Mapping the distortion as a function of the angle (θ) between the observer (*O*) and the velocity (*v*) produces a frequency cosine function of changes from the original frequency (*fo*).

tween the *change* in frequency and the motion. This change in frequency we will call the Doppler shift frequency.

Looking at the Doppler shift frequency, *Df*, we have found that it changes with the wave source velocity. As that velocity increases, the change in frequency increases; as that velocity decreases, the change in frequency decreases. This can be expressed as a proportionality

$$Df \propto V \tag{5.2}$$

where *Df* is the Doppler shift frequency, and *V* is the source velocity.

On a more practical level, the greater the velocity of the wave source, the greater the Doppler shift. In the headphones of a simple Doppler device, we can hear an increase in the audio frequency as the blood increases velocity, and a decrease as the blood slows down.

The wave pattern surrounding a moving source shows that the distortion is not symmetrical, either (Fig. 5-4). In the direction of motion, the *change* in frequency is largest and upward. Just opposite to the direction of motion, the change in frequency is equally as large, but downward. Between these two limits is a continuously changing Doppler shift frequency.

If the change in frequency around the source as a function of direction is graphed, it looks like a trigonometric function (Fig. 5-4). In fact, it traces out the cosine function of an angle. Our proportionality now becomes

$$Df \propto V \cos \theta \tag{5.3}$$

where θ is the "look angle" between the velocity of the object, *V*, and the line between the observer and the source.

V is still the velocity of the source, but $\cos \theta$ introduces a geometric factor. The combined term $V \cos \theta$, is the projection of the source velocity, *V*, onto the connecting line (Fig. 5-5). In other words, $V \cos \theta$ is the closing velocity between source and observer, which is the rate these two are approaching or retreating from one another.

In reviewing our basic events, a good question we might ask is whether or not the Doppler shift frequency is sensitive to the stationary wave frequency. Examination of Doppler shift frequencies from two different sources moving at the same velocity but emitting different frequencies shows that a sensitivity to frequency does exist (Fig.

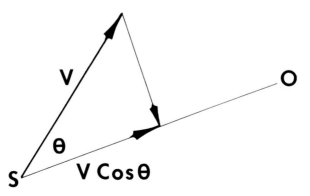

Figure 5-5   Formation of the closing velocity. The terms *V cos* θ in the Doppler equation form the closing velocity. *S* is the wave source, *V* is the source velocity, *O* is the observer, and θ is the angle between the velocity and the line connecting the source and observer.

5-6): as the stationary wave frequency increases, so does the Doppler shift frequency. We can put that factor, F_0, in our proportionality as well

$$Df \propto F_0 V \cos \theta \qquad (5.4)$$

where F_0 is the stationary wave frequency.

Because the Doppler effect depends upon the propagation velocity of the waves, it is appropriate to ask whether this velocity could also affect the Doppler shift frequency. As it turns out, an increase in wave propagation velocity is accompanied by a decrease in Doppler shift frequency, i.e., an inverse relationship exists between these two.

But why would this be true? The answer lies in the fact that as waves move faster (an increasing propagation velocity), they require a much higher source velocity to get the same amount of wave pattern distortion. Conversely, when waves move more slowly, it is easier for movement to distort them.

The proportionality now looks like

$$Df \propto (F_0/c) V \cos \theta \qquad (5.5)$$

where c is the wave propagation velocity.

This proportionality takes an interesting turn if we insert a new term for the frequency-to-velocity ratio. This term comes from the original wavelength-frequency equation at the beginning of this chapter. The frequency-to-velocity ratio in the Doppler relationship becomes the reciprocal of the stationary frequency wave length

$$1/\lambda_0 = F_0/c \qquad (5.6)$$

where λ_0 is the stationary frequency wavelength. Substituting this term in the proportionality yields

$$Df \propto (V \cos \theta) / \lambda_0. \qquad (5.7)$$

This relationship shows clearly that the Doppler shift frequency depends upon the ratio of the closing velocity ($V \cos \theta$) and the stationary wave length (λ_0). The Doppler shift frequency will increase with decreasing wavelength because the closing velocity has a proportionally greater effect on the wavelength.

Although these influences are more difficult to visualize as part of the first Doppler effect, they do occur. A detailed mathematical approach would show the same sort of proportionality we just arrived at for the second Doppler effect. Producing the final Doppler equation for ultrasound, however, requires the combination of both Doppler effects.

Combining the Two Doppler Effects

In ultrasound applications of Doppler, the red blood cell (RBC) plays a double role. It is first an "observer" of a stationary ultrasound field. Second, the RBC acts as a wave

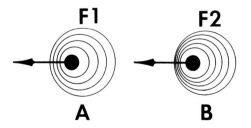

Figure 5-6   The Doppler effect with changing transmitting frequency. By increasing the transmitting frequency, the same velocity produces a greater Doppler shift. Sources *A* and *B* are moving at the same velocity, but *F2* is a higher frequency (smaller wavelength) than *F1*.

source when the waves scatter from its surface. These two physical situations clearly represent the first and second Doppler effects.

The ultrasound field comes from a stationary transducer, and as the waves travel, they establish a stationary ultrasonic field. As the RBC travels through this field, it "sees" a change in ultrasound frequency as a function of its speed and direction of motion.

As the RBC and the ultrasonic waves interact, the waves scatter off the RBC's surface. If the RBC is moving, these reflected waves distort as if the cell were a moving wave source. This represents the second Doppler effect, but the frequency it changes is not the frequency of the stationary system, rather it is the frequency produced by the first Doppler effect. The final effect, then, is the combination of the first and second Doppler effects. The result is the Doppler equation we commonly use in ultrasound

$$Df = 2\,(F_0/c)V\cos\theta \tag{5.8}$$

The number 2 comes from the combination of these two Doppler effects.

Examining the two Doppler effects shows that although they seem to be the same, they are not. Although relative motion between the source of waves and an observer may appear independent of who is moving, the symmetry is not perfect. These two effects differ in terms of real and apparent wavelength changes. In the first Doppler effect, the moving receiver perceives a change in frequency, but a stationary receiver sees no change in the waves. The second Doppler effect, however, produces a very real distortion in the wave pattern that would be witnessed by either a moving or stationary observer. Thus, although these two effects look mathematically alike, one is real and the other is only apparent.

Using the Tool

Without some idea about what is happening to each of the elements in an equation, it is hard to convert it into an effective tool. Looking at each of the elements in the Doppler equation gives some insight about: 1) what will be measured in Doppler signal processing; 2) what must be controlled to make the equation work; 3) what must be assumed about the tissue-ultrasound interaction; and 4) what we are ultimately trying to understand.

Understanding and measuring flow is really a matter of determining the absolute velocities of the RBCs. From the original Doppler equation

$$Df = 2\,(F_0/c)\,V\cos\theta \tag{5.8}$$

we solve for velocity, which produces

$$V = (Df\,c)/(2\,F_0\cos\theta) \tag{5.9}$$

Considering this equation from the viewpoint of ultrasound technology, the following situations will emerge. First, the Doppler shift frequency, Df, will be measured in the sonograph via a circuit that detects the Doppler shift frequency by comparing the returning echo signal with the transmitted signal. Second, the velocity of propagation, c, will be designated as 1,540 m/s, the soft tissue average. Third, the Doppler sonograph will control the transmit frequency, F_0, which establishes a known source frequency for the traveling ultrasound. Within the device, F_0 will also serve as a reference to detect the Doppler shift frequency.

The angle θ will be the most difficult variable to control. Knowing the Doppler angle permits a calculation of cos θ, removing the remaining unknown in the Doppler equation. In general, cos θ changes very slowly from 0° to 20°. Table 5-1 shows how this function changes near 0°, 60°, and 80°. And, of course, as cos θ approaches 1, that is when the motion is completely along the connecting line, the Doppler shift frequency is at maximum. Thus, to assure accuracy in velocity calculations used in echocardiography, a sonographer tries to keep the Doppler angle close to 0° by selecting views that parallel the flow of interest.[5] Because many of the major arteries and veins of interest are parallel or nearly parallel to the skin, a standard angle of 60° is most often used for vessels.[6]

In pulsed-Doppler systems, the ability to depict high Doppler shift frequencies encounters an upper limit determined by how often the system samples motion (the pulse repetition frequency). This sampling limit is called the *Nyquist frequency*. When *Df* exceeds the Nyquist frequency, a phenomenon called high-frequency aliasing occurs, which prevents an accurate measurement of the maximum Doppler shift frequency when conventional analytical techniques are in use.[7] Although aliasing is treated in more detail in Chapter 8, we are currently interested in the solutions to aliasing offered by the Doppler equation.

The Doppler equation suggests two alternatives to the ceiling imposed by the Nyquist limit. The first alternative is to lower the transmit frequency. This does not change the Nyquist limit but instead repositions the aliasing Doppler shift frequency below it. The second alternative is to change the Doppler angle, θ, to a more obtuse value (closer to 90°), which lowers *Df* below the Nyquist limit. In this manner, the Doppler equation shows not only the variables that influence the Doppler effect, but also some strategies for keeping the range of Doppler shift frequencies appropriate for analysis.

Obtuse Doppler angles can create other problems, however. As the angle between the vessel and the transducer approaches 90° all Doppler shift frequencies decrease. In this situation, low frequencies that may be part of diastolic flow or attenuated systolic velocities (a long, tight stenosis) will disappear. Without thinking about the Doppler angle influence, a clinician might approach a vessel too steeply, fail to hear the Doppler sounds, and judge the vessel to be occluded. This is not an uncommon error.

Table 5-1.   Changes in Cosine Values

Angle (degrees)	Value
0	1.000
5	0.996
15	0.966
20	0.940
55	0.574
60	0.500
65	0.423
75	0.259
80	0.174
85	0.087
89	0.018

More About the Doppler Angle and Flow Velocity

For several very good reasons, Doppler ultrasound users have a growing interest in moving away from the Doppler shift frequency to blood velocity as an expression of flow events. At the outset, blood flow velocity is more physiological. It seems to have a strong connection to clinical events such as predicting the failure of a bypass graft.[8] Furthermore, expressing velocity does not require additional information such as the Doppler angle and transmit frequency. In addition, velocity information is the first step in calculating volume flow through a vessel or the heart, using a spatial average velocity over the flow lumen. Clearly, expressing Doppler information in terms of blood flow velocities is more representative of circulatory events and facilitates further quantitation. Considering what is already known about hemodynamic events, a caution flag should immediately go up when velocity is blindly offered as a substitute for a measured Doppler shift frequency.

Calculating a velocity is easier when the ultrasound beam is nearly parallel to the flow vector or when we have a clear view of the flow streamlines using color flow imaging. In the parallel flow situation, the Doppler-angle uncertainty has minimal effect. But if we lack visual information about the direction of flow streamlines, how do we quantitate flow velocities in the vascular system, where Doppler angles deviate markedly from 0° to 180°? This, in turn, leads to the question: How much do we really know about the geometry of flow within a vascular lumen?

The first indication that events within the vascular system are more complex than expected comes from the observation that velocity calculations disperse more than frequency measurements alone. Another piece of evidence is the observation that upstream Doppler shift frequencies often differ markedly from downstream frequencies when recorded from the same point. If blood motion were parallel to the vessel walls, the frequencies would be the same. Finally, an uncomfortable number of false positives still occur with duplex systems.

The most direct evidence, however, comes from color flow imaging and angiodynography. These imaging techniques provide a real-time picture of vascular events, portraying the tissue in gray scale and blood flow in color. Images from these systems clearly show that: 1) flow is never axial in a curving vessel; 2) flow can be very nonaxial even in straight vessels; 3) plaques are clearly not positioned symmetrically within vessels; and 4) jets produced by these lesions are not necessarily axial to the vessel lumen. The assumption that flow is always axial and parallel to the vessel walls is assuredly not a good one, despite the fact that it was all we had for a while. This lack of flow symmetry often explains the difficulty of showing that some individuals are indeed normal, despite Doppler events suggesting vascular disease.

Ultimately, the individual sample volume used by all duplex systems is blind and inarticulate, unable to express the angle at which blood flow enters and leaves it. That means it is the responsibility of the operator to determine the real Doppler angle and include this angle in any velocity calculations. Determining the real Doppler angle may require some careful mapping using the sample volume to find out how the major streamline points within the vessel lumen. Imaging the blood flow within the vascular compartment, however, can reveal these otherwise invisible vascular events.

Figure 5-7 is an angiodynogram of nonaxial flow through a carotid artery (see color section between pp. 116 and 117). Figure 5-8 shows how a nonaxial flow pattern can produce a situation in which upstream Doppler shift frequencies are much higher

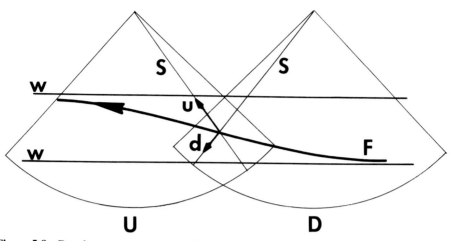

Figure 5-8   Doppler measurement errors due to nonaxial flow geometry. When a major streamline (*F*) moves from the one side of a vessel wall to the other, upstream measurements (*u*) will be higher because the Doppler angle is less than downstream (*d*). *S* is the sample line, *U* and *D* are up- and downstream sectors, respectively, and *w* indicates the vessel walls.

than the downstream measurements. This particular error comes from the diagonal flow pattern that crosses the vascular lumen.

Some Final Thoughts

Converting Doppler shift frequencies into velocities seems rather direct: simply determine the parameters of the Doppler equation and plug in the values. Most sonographs and duplex machines, however, have a limit on placing the Doppler angle cursor. Angle readout values typically change in 1° steps. As a result, an angle correction is in reality ± 1°. How large a role can this 1° uncertainty play in velocity calculations?

Table 5-2 shows how a 1° error changes the velocity calculation for several Doppler angles. As the Doppler angle approaches 60°, the error is only 3% per degree. At 80°,

Table 5-2.   Error Rates for Velocity Calculations for Various Doppler Angles

Angle (degrees)	Percent error/degree
0	0.015
5	0.167
15	0.482
20	0.650
55	2.5
60	3.0
65	3.8
75	6.5
80	9.9
85	20.0
88	50.0
89	100.0

however, the error grows to 10% per degree, and rapidly accelerates as the angle approaches 90°. Clearly, to make the best estimates of velocities, Doppler angles must be less than 80°.

Because of the angle dependence in velocity calculations, often the best approach is to change the scanning window. Transcranial Doppler imaging and echocardiography are good examples of this process. By selecting the right scanning windows into the cranium, the cerebral arteries are often very close to a 0° angle. As a result, estimates of velocity have proven valuable in detecting cerebral spasm after subarachnoid hemorrhage[9] and estimating pressure gradients in cardiac outflow obstructions.[10] And all of it is based on the Doppler equation.

References

1. White, DN. Johann Christian Doppler and his effect—A brief history. *Ultrasound Med Biol* 8: 583–591, 1982.
2. Mihalas, D, and Routly, PM. *Galactic Astronomy.* San Francisco: WH Freeman and Co, 1968, pp 12, 31.
3. Hussey, M. *Diagnostic Ultrasound: An Introduction to the Interactions Between Ultrasound and Biological Tissues.* London: Blackie & Son, 1975, p 38.
4. Parry, RJ, and Chivers, RC. Data of the velocity and attenuation of ultrasound in mammalian tissues—A survey. *In* Linzer, M (ed): *Ultrasonic Tissue Characterization II,* National Bureau of Standards Special Publication 525. Washington, DC: US Government Printing Office, 1979, pp 343–360.
5. Richards, KL, Cannon, SR, Crawford, MH, et al. Noninvasive diagnosis of aortic and mitral valve disease with pulsed-Doppler spectral analysis. *Am J Cardiol* 51:1122–1127, 1983.
6. Roederer, GO, Langlois, Y, and Strandness, DE, Jr. Comprehensive noninvasive evaluation of extracranial cerebrovascular disease. *In* Hershey, FB, Barnes, RW, and Sumner, DS (eds): *Noninvasive Diagnosis of Vascular Disease.* Pasadena, California: Appleton Davies, 1984, pp 177–216.
7. Hatle, L, and Angelsen, B. *Doppler Ultrasound in Cardiology.* Philadelphia: Lea & Febiger, 1982, p 51.
8. Bandyk, DF, Cato, RF, and Towne, JB. A low flow velocity predicts failure of femoropopliteal and femorotibial bypass grafts. *Surgery* 98:799–809, 1985.
9. Lindegaard, KF, Normes, H, Bakke, JS, et al. Cerebral vasospasm after subarachnoid haemorrhage investigated by means of transcranial Doppler ultrasound. *Acta Neurosurg* 42 (Suppl):81–84, 1988.
10. Lima, CO, Sahn, DJ, Valdes-Cruz, LM, et al. Prediction of the severity of left ventricular outflow tract obstruction by quantitative two-dimensional echocardiographic Doppler Studies. *Circulation* 68:348–354, 1983.

6

Primary Steps in Doppler Signal Processing

From developing the Doppler equation, we learned that motion information does not reside within the absolute frequency but rather the change in frequency of returning echoes. This change in frequency is the Doppler shift frequency and represents the result of the Doppler effect. As a consequence, signal processing steps within any Doppler system will focus on separating the Doppler shift frequency from the returning echo signals. The changing character of the Doppler shift frequencies over time will depict blood motion.

Two primary forms of Doppler operating modes offer different methods of obtaining the Doppler shift frequency: continuous wave (CW), and pulsed wave or pulsed Doppler. We first concentrate on the CW Doppler system to understand how to obtain the Doppler shift frequency. This model also illustrates the sources of the signal mix in the system output. From this position, the next step examines the pulsed Doppler system in terms of the basic Doppler goals of source, form, frequency, and direction. These goals ultimately provide organization and meaning to the essential steps in Doppler signal processing.

CW Doppler System

The term "continuous wave" describes a transmitting and receiving process in which the transmitter and receiver is on continuously. In Doppler ultrasound, this means the system continuously and simultaneously transmits and receives ultrasound signals.

Typically, continuous transmission and reception of ultrasound involves two separate transducers, one for generating ultrasound, the other for receiving the echoes. But two transducers are not absolutely necessary; a single transducer could also do the job.[1] A common transducer, however, would require the returning echoes to be superimposed on a very large transmission signal within the transducer. Separating signals with such a difference in amplitude is a very difficult engineering problem. As a result, CW systems almost uniformly use two separate transducers. Despite a two-transducer organization, signals from the receiving transducer will still contain strong signals from stationary echo sources in the transmitting beam. These strong signals are mixed together with the much smaller signals from the moving RBCs within the vessels.

Because uniform transducer characteristics make a CW system work better, the two transducers are often halves of the same wafer-shaped parent transducer. The single transducer is simply split and mounted in a common housing.[2]

Most of these transducers are undamped (they vibrate naturally for a long period of time). They also have relatively narrow bandwidths (transmit only a narrow range of frequencies) and have higher quality-factor (called Q by engineers, which means less energy becomes heat inside the transducer) than typical imaging transducers.[3] These Doppler transducers are cut to very specific frequencies and are electronically matched to the system transmitter. Such conditions are quite opposite to the needs of a typical imaging transducer. This contrast in needs compromises performance later when we consider using the same transducer for both imaging and Doppler in a duplex system.

Continuous transmission means that a CW system loses the ability to determine uniquely the range of various echo sources within the ultrasound beam. The source of the echo signals remains to be determined, and designing the transducer in a CW system to operate over a specific region can help satisfy this need. For example, canting the two transducer elements toward one another will overlap the transmitting and receiving ultrasound beams. The area of overlap, called the region of maximum sensitivity, helps limit contributing echo sources to a small region in space. Increasing the transducer frequency can limit this region further with better focusing and limited penetration from tissue attenuation.

Signal Processing Organization

As in any ultrasound system, signal processing begins with the transducer. Here the transducer converts the electrical energy from the transmitter into an ultrasound field. At the same time, the receiving transducer converts the returning echo signals into electrical signals for signal processing.

The design needs of a simple CW Doppler system are not very great. Processing begins with the production of ultrasound by exciting the transducer into vibration. The vibration comes from the mechanical response of the transducer to a varying electrical signal applied across a piezoelectric material. The source of the exciting energy is a master oscillator operating at the transducer natural frequency (Fig. 6-1). Because the transducer has a natural resonant frequency that is the same as the master oscillator frequency, the driving voltage for the transmitter can be very small. For example, a driving voltage can be 10 to 60 V.[3] Furthermore, the normally undamped characteristic of the transducer (its ability to vibrate for a long time with little electrical stimulation) results in relatively high electrical efficiency.

Echoes arise in the tissue and return to the receiving transducer. Dominating the returning echoes are very strong signals from stable, nonmoving, specular echo sources. These louder signals constitute what is called the system leakage signal.[1] Mixed among these very large signals are the much smaller Doppler signals from the moving tissue components and the RBCs.

An effective way of relating these two sorts of signals, the leakage signals and the Doppler signals, is through a phaser diagram (Fig. 6-2). This diagram shows the timing (phase) and amplitude of the returning echo signals. The reference for comparison is the transmitted signal. In this diagram, the main leakage signal becomes a large unmoving vector. This signal has a fixed time relationship with respect to the transmitted

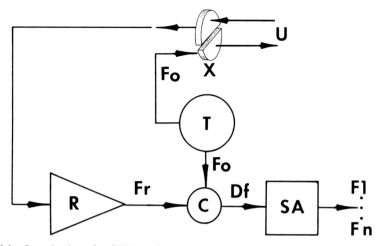

Figure 6-1   Organization of a CW Doppler system. The transducer (*X*) is a split single element, continuously transmitting and receiving ultrasound (*U*). The transmitter (*T*) sends the carrier frequency (*Fo*) to the transducer and to the comparator (*C*). The receiver (*R*) amplifies the return signals (*Fr*), which are compared with *Fo* to produce the Doppler signal (*Df*). This signal goes to a spectral analysis stage (*SA*), producing a set of frequency components, *F1* to *Fn*.

signal, i.e., it is not moving. Added to this large vector are the smaller Doppler signals that are changing with RBC motion. They appear as a much smaller vector that adds to the leakage signal. This means the small RBC signals rotate about the end of the larger signal over time. The task is to remove the large, unchanging signal and deal only with the smaller signals representing RBC motion.

The next stage in the signal processing is to amplify the received signals for later processing. A radio frequency (RF) amplifier handles this job (Fig. 6-1). The amplifier stage is usually a logarithmic amplifier. These circuits accept a very large range of input signals and compress them into a smaller, more manageable range (Fig. 6-3).

This nonlinear amplifying technique reduces the input signal dynamic range. At the same time, it also brings the large and small signal amplitudes closer together at the output. As a result, separation of these signals based on amplitude alone requires a nonlinear and sensitive approach.

After signal compression, the system then compares the received and transmitted signals. This occurs at a circuit called a comparator (Fig. 6-1). The comparator can be as simple as a frequency mixing system that beats the transmitted and received signals against one another. The output from such a circuit contains four frequencies: the two individual input frequencies, the sum of the two, and the difference between the two.[4] The difference is, of course, the Doppler shift frequency. The other frequencies are not needed, so they are filtered out.

The comparator can also be a phase-sensing circuit that examines the change in phase of the received signal relative to the transmitted signal.[5] The quadrature phase detector is such a circuit. It produces the Doppler shift frequency as an output.

Because of the range of velocities common to the body and the ultrasound frequencies in use, typical Doppler shift frequencies fall within the human audio spectrum of 20 to 20,000 Hz. As a result, the first Doppler signal analyzer was the human auditory system: people simply listened to the Doppler sounds. This display form is still part of even the most advanced duplex systems available. Every current Doppler system has Doppler sounds going to speakers or headphones.

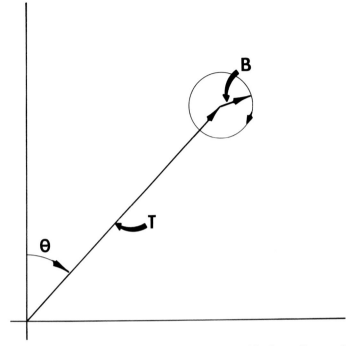

Figure 6-2   Simultaneous reception of blood and tissue signals. This phaser diagram shows the large leakage signal (*T*) from the tissue added to the much smaller blood signals (*B*). Amplitude is indicated by the length of the arrow and direction by θ. The small *circle* shows how the blood signals change phase angle over time, with the vector tip following the small circle.

Doppler signal analysis is not limited to the human auditory system, however. Techniques available to analyze Doppler shift frequencies include the multifilter analyzer, the zero-crossing detector, the autocorrelator, and the fast Fourier transform (FFT) device. (See Chapter 7 for detailed discussions.) After Doppler signal analysis, the signals might appear on a cathode ray tube or a strip chart recorder.

The central question here, however, is not what steps happen to go into frequency analysis, but why frequency analysis is needed at all. The answer to this question lies in the character of the Doppler shift signals and their sources.

Source of the Doppler Signal Mix

A CW Doppler system receiving echoes from a vessel with moving blood does not produce a single tone. Instead, the output is a complex set of many signals, superimposed to form a final signal mix. An oscilloscope placed on the audio output from a Doppler system shows a very complicated wave form (Fig. 6-4) in which individual frequencies are hidden. Such a result should prompt the question: Just what is the source and character of such a complex Doppler signal? The answer will come from building the Doppler output signal from a limited number of echo sources.

Consider first a single echo source moving within the ultrasound field at constant velocity (Figure 6-5, A). This moving solitary reflector produces a single signal with a fixed amplitude and frequency. We can show this signal on a diagram by graphing amplitude on the Y-axis and frequency on the X-axis. The result is a single vertical line

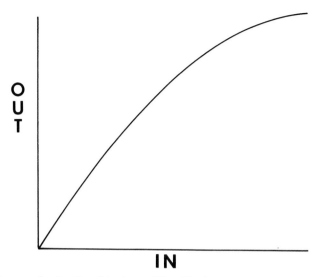

Figure 6-3   Compression in a logarithmic amplifier. The logarithm is an exponential function that changes more slowly than the numbers it represents. In an amplifier, this relationship permits a wide range of input signals (*IN*) to be compressed into a small range at the output (*OUT*). In this case, the output signal is the logarithm of the input signal.

with a fixed amplitude. The reflector motion (velocity) determines the frequency. At the same time, the reflectivity of the echo source determines the signal amplitude.

Adding a second echo source with the same reflectivity and moving with the same velocity as the first changes the result (Figure 6-5, B). The second signal is identical to the first because the motion and reflection conditions are the same. The result is different, however, because these two signals add together, following the rules for the superposition of waves. The new signal has the same frequency as the first, but twice the original amplitude. In other words, the two original signals add together to form a new third signal.

The properties of superimposing waves become central here. The original waves add together in a simple fashion to form a new resultant wave. Importantly, the individual waves that contributed to the result have not lost their own identity.[6] By applying the

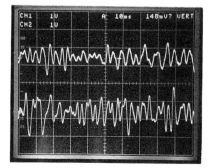

Figure 6-4   Raw audio Doppler signals. Prior to processing with an FFT device, the Doppler signals are a sum of all the individual waves. In this oscilloscope display, signals from the radial artery are on the *top* trace, with signals from the radial vein on the *bottom* trace. The lower trace appears to have more low frequencies; otherwise the two traces are not markedly different. The distinctive flow pattern of artery and vein appears after FFT processing.

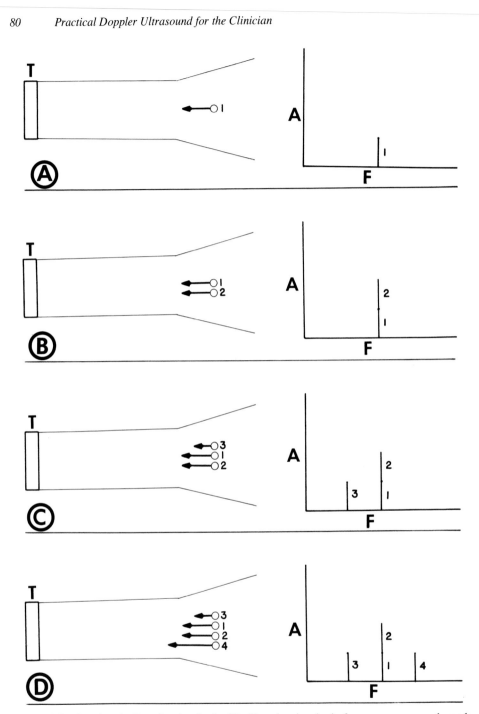

Figure 6-5 Creating the Doppler signal mix. The Doppler signal mix from many sources depends upon the simple superposition of waves. **A,** A single moving echo source (*1*) in an ultrasound beam generated by a transducer (*T*) makes a signal of fixed amplitude (*A*) and frequency (*F*). **B,** A second identical echo source (*2*) moving the same way produces a second signal identical to the first, and they add together (*1 + 2*). **C,** A third, slower echo source makes a new signal, *3,* with a constant amplitude but lower frequency. **D,** A fourth, faster echo source produces another frequency component (*4*) with a higher frequency but constant amplitude. This superposition principle produces the signal mix typical of moving blood, where signal component amplitude is related to the number of RBCs moving the same way.

right operator, these two waves, and indeed any other component waves, could be separated out from the resulting signal.[7]

Let's now add in another echo source, but one moving at a slower velocity (Fig. 6-5, C). The new signal, like the earlier echo signals, will have the same amplitude, but its frequency will be lower because the reflector is moving more slowly. This new wave adds to the other two to produce an even more complex summation. The rules of superposition still apply, and employing the right analysis will again recover this component.

Adding another echo source that is moving faster complicates the output even further (Figure 6-5, D). In this instance, the new component signal has the same amplitude but a higher frequency because its source motion is faster. As before, this new signal also adds to the total signal mix.

Building this signal mix from the individual reflectors provides a view of how various echo signals contribute to form a spectrum. Just looking at the summed output signals is not enough. We need a spectrum that shows the components in terms of frequency and amplitude. The range of spectral frequencies, of course, shows the range of velocities of the targets. The amplitude of each frequency component, in turn, represents the number of targets moving along together at the same velocity. Thus, examining the spectral output from a vessel carrying RBCs will reveal the range of RBC velocities within the ultrasound beam. In addition, the frequency component amplitudes show how many of the RBCs are moving together. This sort of analysis is shown in Figure 6-6.

Such a spectral relationship has other considerations as well. For example, what might happen if the ultrasound beam were pointed at a small, high-velocity jet of blood? Based on the model we have created, a physically small jet would limit the number of RBCs entering the ultrasound beam. Fewer cells in the beam means smaller echo amplitudes and, thereby, smaller Doppler frequency component amplitudes. It follows then, that small, high-velocity jets may be difficult to detect, not because of their high Doppler frequencies, but because they simply lack signal strength. It is a problem that can decrease the ability of a Doppler system to separate a 99% carotid stenosis from an occlusion.

In both CW and pulsed Doppler systems, RBCs moving at different velocities in different directions produce a wide range of Doppler frequencies. In contrast, cells moving together in like fashion produce a much narrower range of Doppler frequencies. Thus, diseases or conditions that change the organization of flow also change the range of Doppler shift frequencies. Indeed, the spread in frequencies can indicate the amount of disease present in a vascular compartment. The task of any analysis system,

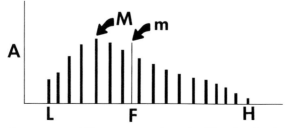

Figure 6-6 The mode frequency within a spectrum. A graph of Doppler signal amplitude (*A*) versus frequency (*F*) may not be symmetrical. In this case, *M* is the mode frequency with the greatest amplitude. The mean frequency (*m*) is different from the mode frequency because the spectrum is asymmetrical. *L* is the lowest frequency; *H*, the highest.

then, is to separate the complicated sum of signals at the Doppler detector output into component frequencies that will let us examine the details of blood flow within the ultrasound beam. For example, from these separations come measurements of peak systolic frequencies and the spectral broadening that are classical Doppler signs of vascular disease.

The output from a typical CW Doppler system can show how the form and frequency content of complex Doppler signals change over time. The system may even provide basic information about direction of flow relative to the transducer. It will lack, however, the spatial resolution needed to determine explicitly the source of echo signals, i.e., where they come from. A unique determination of the echo source is provided by the other side of the Doppler coin: the pulsed Doppler system.

In addition to the lack of spatial information there is a very tough signal separation problem for CW systems. A CW Doppler ultrasound beam integrates all signals, both stationary tissue and moving blood. Typically, the signals used to follow moving blood have a size only 1% that of the larger tissue signal amplitudes. In general, a pulsed-Doppler system limits the echo signal sources and, as a result, improves the signal-to-noise ratio.

Improving Spatial Resolution with a Pulsed-Doppler System

Although a pulsed-Doppler system asks the same questions about events within the vascular compartments as does a CW system, it uses different techniques. These techniques provide a new level of information but not without some problems and limitations.

Like any echo-ranging technique, pulsed Doppler cycles between transmitting and receiving. Initially, the system sends out a burst of ultrasound and waits for the returning echoes. The system does not process all of the returning echoes, however. Instead, the receiver counts time until the signals from a specific location arrive at the transducer. When these echoes arrive, the receiver turns on and processes the echo signals for Doppler shift frequencies, then turns off again. This process of narrowing the receiver function to a specific range is called range gating.[5]

Range gating provides primary spatial information about the source of the Doppler signals. Common to both the pulsed-Doppler and advanced CW systems is processing to determine signal form, frequency content, and direction. Figure 6-7 shows a schematic representation of both CW and pulsed-Doppler techniques.

Controlled Transmission

Any ultrasound signal-processing system is powerless to extract information about the phase and frequency of the received echo if the character of the transmitted signal is unknown. The first step with a pulsed-Doppler system, then, is to fix the phase (timing) and frequency of the transmitted burst of ultrasound.[8] Fixing the transmitted signal phase and frequency makes the system "coherent." The organization of a coherent pulsed Doppler system is shown in Fig. 6-8.

The internal reference for frequency and phase comes from a master oscillator (MO) circuit within the system (Fig. 6-8). The MO oscillates at the same frequency as the transducer. For example, a 5-MHz Doppler transducer would have a 5-MHz MO frequency. Because the MO is a fundamental reference within the system, the circuit

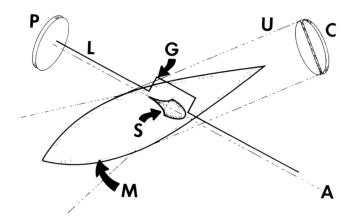

Figure 6-7 Sampling fields for the pulsed and CW Doppler systems. The pulsed Doppler (*P*) transmits a burst of ultrasound to create the sample volume (*S*). The signal is localized using the receiver range gate (*G*), which opens the receiver for processing when signals from this range arrive at the transducer. *L* is the time line and *A* is the ultrasound beam axis. The CW Doppler system (*C*) points the two portions of the transducer toward each other to make a region of maximum sensitivity (*M*). *U* is the ultrasound beam.

design stresses frequency stability despite changing power supply voltages or operating temperature.

One of the signal outputs from the MO goes to a frequency divider. This circuit accepts a signal input at one frequency and produces an output signal of a lower frequency, called a subharmonic of the input signal. Because the output signal is subharmonic, it is an exact submultiple of the input signal. For example, a 5-MHz MO frequency might be divided down 1,000 times to produce an output frequency of 5,000 Hz. This output signal becomes the pulse repetition frequency (PRF) for the system.

The PRF is the number of times each second the system goes through its pulse-listen cycle. PRFs in pulsed-Doppler systems can range from as low as 1,000 Hz to as high as 20,000 Hz. In general, the design of the system will match the PRF to the distance it will show in the image (image depth) and the highest Doppler shift frequency it expects to detect. As the display depth increases, the PRF decreases because the ultrasound propagation velocity is fixed at 1,540 m/s.

On a more practical basis, the actual division value matches the system's field of view. Typically, shorter fields of view will have higher PRFs. To maintain the highest Doppler signal resolution, a system selects the highest possible PRF based on the maximum display depth at any time. For example, a PRF of 5,000 Hz would match a maximum depth range of 14.8 cm. The relationship between PRF and the MO frequencies is shown in Fig. 6-9.

The output signal from the frequency divider controls a gated transmitter circuit (Fig. 6-8). The gated transmitter, in turn, generates a time window for another MO signal output. This window opens on cue from the frequency divider and closes after a fixed number of half-cycles. The gate, then, could define a window that is two, three, or any number of cycles long. In this manner, the gated transmitter generates a driving signal for the transducer. With the excitation coming from the gated transmitter, the transducer vibration always starts at the same time in the MO wave train and ends a fixed number of half-cycles later. The result is a burst of ultrasound with a known phase and frequency (a coherent signal).

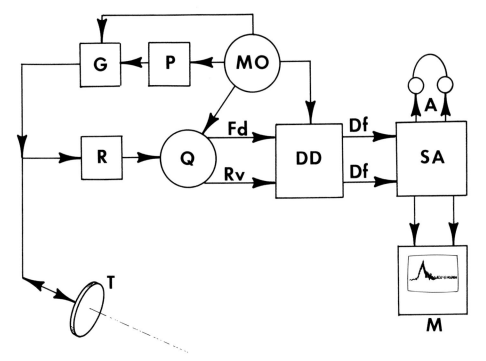

Figure 6-8   The coherent pulsed Doppler system. *T* is the transducer. *MO* is the master oscillator, *P* is the pulse repetition frequency divider, *G* is the gated transmitter. *R* is the receiver, and *Q* is the quadrature phase detector, creating forward (*Fd*) and reverse (*Rv*) channels that go to the Doppler detector (*DD*). The forward and reverse Doppler frequencies (*Df*) then go to a spectrum analyzer (*SA*) and split into two display forms: audio (*A*, also shown by headphones) or spectral display on a monitor (*M*). See the text for operating details.

The output from the gated transmitter excites the transducer into vibration at the frequency and phase determined entirely by the driving voltage. This transfer of energy should be high fidelity, i.e., the transducer should introduce no changes in either the phase or frequency of the ultrasound that leaves the transducer.

In a pulsed-Doppler duplex system, both Doppler and imaging modes use the same transducer. In general, an imaging transducer is highly damped, which produces a broad frequency band width. If the band width is large enough, the system can use the same transducer to image on one frequency and handle Doppler signals on another. Such a dual operation is hardly ideal because the imaging mode will operate more efficiently than the Doppler mode.

The Receiver

After transduction, the returning echo signals go to the system receiver. The system receiver or RF amplifier (Fig. 6-8) has two primary purposes. First, it amplifies the echo signals up to a voltage that permits further signal processing. Second, it provides a range-gating function that limits the source of the echo signals to a specific range from the transducer.

The RF amplifier is usually the first site for signal processing beyond amplification. The input dynamic range for the Doppler signals can easily exceed 100 dB for very deep vessels.[9] This is an almost impossible task for the RF amplifier. It must accept and

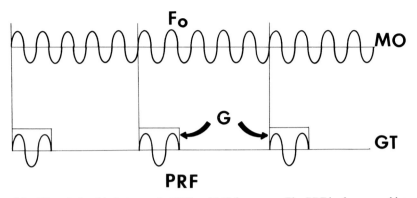

Figure 6-9   The relationship between the PRF and MO frequency. The *PRF* is always a subharmonic of the *MO* frequency (*Fo*). The gated transmitter (*GT*) opens up for a short duration (*G*), permitting a fixed number of cycles to reach the transducer.

amplify a range of signals that exceeds 100,000:1. Applying time-gain compensation or TGC to the RF amplifier, however, can reduce the signal range to a more realistic level. In addition, the smaller range of signals fits more easily within the operating ranges of the subsequent quadrature phase detector, Doppler detector, and frequency analysis devices.

Quadrature Phase Detector

As an echo source moves, the phase of the returning echo signals changes. These changes in phase relative to the MO signal provide two pieces of information. First, a changing phase indicates that an echo source is moving. Second, how the phase changes indicates the direction of that motion relative to the transducer. Such phase changes are decoded by the quadrature phase-detector circuit (Fig. 6-8).

We can see how motion information is derived from the phase of an echo signal by examining the timing relationships between an echo signal from a moving source and the MO signal (Fig. 6-10). First, let's consider the MO signal with time advancing from left to right. As echo signals arrive from an echo source moving toward the transducer, these echo signals advance in time, moving to the left. On the other hand, were the echo source moving away from the transducer, the echo signals would regress in time, moving to the right. The quadrature phase detector is sensitive to such changes, separating the signals into directional output channels based on these phase changes.

The quadrature phase detector has two signal inputs, one from the MO and the other from the echo signal. The phase detector output consists of two signals, one representing motion toward the transducer (the forward channel) and the other representing motion away from the transducer (the reverse channel).

These two output channels look the same. They both have RF signals, but the phase or time relationship between the two channels is a function of the direction of echo source motion. For example, if the echo source motion is toward the transducer, then the forward output channel *leads* the reverse channel by 90°. On the other hand, if the echo source motion is away from the transducer, then the forward channel *lags* the reverse channel by 90° .

On a technical level, the two directional channels are also known by their phase relationship. The forward channel is the "in-phase" or I channel. The reverse channel,

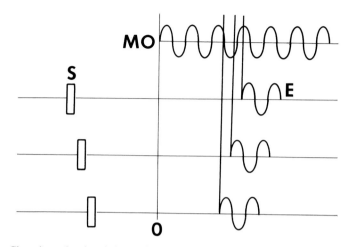

Figure 6-10   Changing echo signal phase with echo source motion. *0* is the transducer face with time to the right of the line and range to the left of the line. As the echo source (*S*) moves, the echo signal (*E*) changes timing (phase) with respect to the MO signal (*MO*). Movement closer to the transducer moves the echo signal to the left. Movement away from the transducer moves the echo signal to the right.

on the other hand, is often called the "quadrature" or Q channel because it is 90° out of phase with the other channel.

After this separation of events into forward and reverse channels, the signals are ready for Doppler shift frequency detection.

Doppler Detector

The primary function of a Doppler detector is to extract the Doppler shift frequency from the RF signals in both forward and reverse channels. Within each of these channels, the RF signals can hold stationary and moving echo signals. This last step in getting the Doppler shift frequency depends upon the phase relationships between the forward and reverse channels and the MO signal (Fig. 6-8). The goal is to obtain two audio channels containing Doppler shift signals that represent motion toward and away from the transducer.

Because the frequency change in any single echo signal is so small with respect to the transmitted frequency, a direct frequency measurement of echo signal changes cannot work well.[5] For example, separating a Doppler shift of 500 Hz from an RF frequency of 5,000,500 Hz is not an easy task. On the other hand, a changing phase is again a very sensitive measure of frequency change. Often another phase detector demodulates the changing RF in each channel into a Doppler shift frequency.

The Doppler detector puts out two audio channels, one containing information about motion toward the transducer and the other information about motion away from the transducer. These two channels carry the complete mix of Doppler shift frequencies contained in the returning echo signal and signify both the existence of motion and its direction.

Doppler Signal Analysis

Doppler signal analysis seeks to determine the frequency content of a Doppler signal and how these frequencies change over time. A direct analysis can come from simply listening to the Doppler frequencies. The human auditory system is capable of a very sophisticated pattern analysis that cannot be replicated by machines. Often, then, the two channels of audio information (forward and reverse flow) at the output from the Doppler detector pass in stereo to human ears.

Human auditory analysis can work rather well but requires a lot of training and experience. Teaching this audio analytical skill to others requires a common set of experiences for the teacher and trainee. In addition, interpretation remains very subjective, a fact that slowed the growth of Doppler use for a long time.

New, more objective techniques are now available to make Doppler signal analysis fast and accurate. These techniques, which rely more on visual pattern recognition rather than skillful listening, include multifilter analysis, which assesses the frequency components by filtering for specific frequencies; zero-crossing detectors that respond to the time intervals between signal zero crossings to estimate frequency content; and the fast Fourier transform (FFT) devices that compute Fourier frequency components. These analytical tools are examined in more detail in Chapter 7.

After the Doppler signals are separated into components, they are ready for display. This display should show the range of Doppler shift frequencies present in the output and how the frequencies change over time. The presentation should be able to demonstrate such parameters as the variation of the maximum frequency or mean frequency over time (measurements of form). A display mode should also show which frequencies are present throughout the cardiac cycle (measurement of frequency content). Thus, from transducer to display, Doppler signal processing looks at the source, direction, form, and frequency of the Doppler shift signals (Fig. 6-8). And these are, of course, the primary goals in the application of Doppler ultrasound.

References

1. Baker, DW, Forster, FK, and Daigle, RE. Doppler Principles and Techniques. *In* Fry, FJ (ed): *Ultrasound: Its Applications in Medicine and Biology,* Part 1. New York: Elsevier Scientific, 1978, pp 161–287.
2. Waxham, RD. Doppler ultrasound. *Radiology Today,* April/May 1980.
3. Wells, PNT. *Physical Principles of Ultrasonic Diagnosis.* New York: Academic Press, 1969, pp 197, 200.
4. Orr, WI. *Radio Handbook,* Ed 17. New Augusta, IN: Editors and Engineers, 1967, p 201.
5. Atkinson, P, and Woodcock, JP. *Doppler Ultrasound and Its Use in Clinical Measurement.* New York: Academic Press, 1982, pp 31, 67.
6. Halliday, D, and Resnick, R. *Physics For Students of Science and Engineering.* New York: John Wiley, 1962, p 400.
7. Kreyszig, E. *Advanced Engineering Mathematics.* New York: John Wiley, 1962, pp 464–491.
8. Baker, DW, and Daigle, RE. Noninvasive ultrasonic flowmetry. *In* Hwang, NHC and Normann, NA (eds): *Cardiovascular Flow Dynamics and Measurements.* Baltimore: University Park Press, 1977, pp 151–189.
9. Powis, RL and Powis, WJ. *A Thinker's Guide to Ultrasonic Imaging.* Baltimore: Urban & Schwarzenberg, 1984, pp 203–238.

7

Signal-Processing Details

A Closer Look at the Tools

Chapter 6 provided a basic look at the signal-processing organization in continuous wave (CW) and pulsed-Doppler systems. Although this would be enough information to run most Doppler sonographs, the more advanced Doppler systems require a better understanding to make them work at their full potential. These systems are more complicated because they give the operator more ways to deal with the problems of scanning. Knowing what to do and when to do it requires more than a casual acquaintance with the machine. Along with a few more details about individual signal-processing steps, this chapter examines the strengths and weaknesses of several different processing approaches. We start with the transducers.

Improving the Transducers

Transducers are at the very center of imaging, and the same is true for Doppler ultrasound. How well a transducer works defines success or failure for an ultrasound system. This dependence increases when dealing with the unusually small signals associated with Doppler ultrasound. After the business of making and receiving ultrasound, the next task for even a CW Doppler transducer is to determine the source of the echo signals, i.e., to determine what vessel we are viewing.

Improving the spatial discrimination of a CW system begins by canting the transmitting and receiving transducers toward one another. This overlaps the two transducer beams, creating a region of maximum sensitivity. In a single transducer, the mathematical product of the receiving directivity (receiving beam) width and the transmitting beam width define the effective beam width.[1] As a result, the transducer appears to have a smaller beam width than either of the functional beams alone. This relationship, however, does not hold exactly for a CW transducer because the transmitting beam and receiving beam are not really superimposed.

A designer can narrow both the receiving and transmitting beams in a CW system by focusing the transducer pair. Focusing and canting the two beams from the same transducer markedly narrows the region of sensitivity. The focusing can come from either internal transducer shaping or an external lens. The effective region of maximum sensitivity appears in Figure 7-1.

Another way of improving the spatial resolution of a CW system is to combine a focused transducer pair with a higher operating frequency. At a higher operating frequency, tissue attenuation shortens the sampling zone. Higher frequencies usually also have improved focusing that further narrows the contributing beams (Fig. 7-1). Using the frequency-dependent tissue attenuation in this manner limits the application of CW Doppler to more superficial vessels. Most often, this is where the vascular anatomy is more complex.

Combining CW Doppler with conventional imaging can increase some of the operating limits of this form of duplex system. Putting CW Doppler on conventional transducers is still new: only a few manufacturers have made the attempt to blend these technologies together. Figure 7-2 shows some examples of CW duplex organization.

One method of making the combination work centers on an annular phased array, which consists of a set of concentric transducer rings. Each ring functions as a separate and independent transducer element. The central element in this geometry is usually a single transducer. Splitting the central element into two parts permits CW Doppler operation.

Another combination that works is based on the linear phased array, which comprises a set of individually unfocused transducer elements. Several of these elements can work together electronically to form a pair of CW transducers.

The end of these sorts of innovation is not in sight. Many of the new Doppler systems are approaching the theoretical limits of internal signal processing. As a result, we can expect to see more attention paid to the transducer portion of the signal stream in the future.

Techniques of Range Gating

An obvious difference between CW and pulsed-Doppler systems is the range-gating function of the latter. Range gating limits the system's processing to signals from a region specified by the operator. Determining the source of an echo signal is easier still if the display also shows something about where the range gate sits in the internal anatomy. For this reason, a pulsed-Doppler system usually includes some form of imaging. Early systems combined an M-mode display with Doppler to show the sampling site. Current systems typically use a real time, gray-scale image.

Essential to range gating is the assumption that ultrasound travels in the tissue at

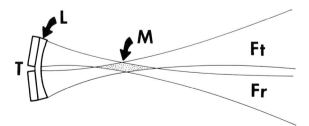

Figure 7-1   Forming the maximum sensitivity region. A CW Doppler limits the signals reaching the system by forming a region of maximum sensitivity (*M*). By separating transducer elements (*T*) and focusing with a lens (*L*), the transmitting field (*Ft*) and receiving field (*Fr*) overlap to form this most sensitive region.

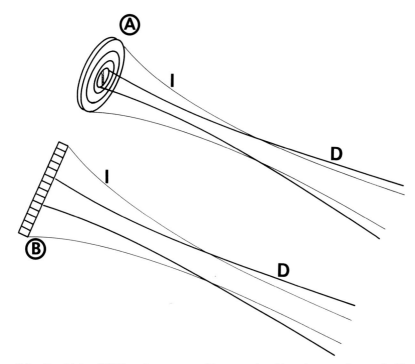

Figure 7-2 Combining CW Doppler systems with conventional imaging transducers. **A,** The annular array can form an imaging beam (*I*) using the transducer rings. At the same time, it can have a CW Doppler transducer in the center, forming a Doppler beam (*D*). **B,** A linear phased array can use central transducers in the same fashion, creating separate imaging (*I*) and Doppler (*D*) beams.

1,540 m/s. In blood, this velocity increases to about 1,580 m/s, a difference that introduces only a small positional error. Knowing the velocity of propagation facilitates timing the ultrasound reception to coincide with the transmitting burst to represent time "zero." Each 13 μs of listening time then represents 1 cm of tissue range.

Counting time from the transmitting burst to the expected arrival time sets the start of the range gate. This time relationship is shown in Figure 7-3. The duration of the gate, on the other hand, is usually the same as the length of the transmitted burst. At the same time, the ultrasound burst length and beam width define the sample volume

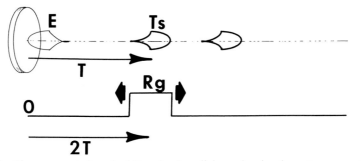

Figure 7-3 The range gate in pulsed Doppler. Localizing echo signals centers on range gating in pulsed Doppler systems. The gate (*Rg*) is a sliding processing window that accepts signals from a specific region. The gate is typically as long as the transmitted burst (*Ts*). Localization depends on a constant velocity. The system computes gate position as twice (*2T*) the one-way propagation time (*T*), starting at time *0*. *E* is the returning echo signal at the transducer.

size. In turn, the sample volume geometry defines the volume of sampled tissue. Matching the length of the range gate to the transmitter sample volume ensures that the combination of the two will not distort the shape of the Doppler signals. Distortions in shape will introduce new frequencies to later spectral analysis.[2]

For all practical purposes, range gating seems to specify a region in space uniquely. This is not true, however, if the system repeats a sampling process (transmitting and receiving) over very short intervals, that is, when the pulse repetition frequency (PRF) becomes very high. If the ultrasound does not die out within the tissue between pulse-listen cycles, reflections from deeper echo sources can reach the receiver when the range gate is open. The result is the range ambiguity artifact.[3] Figure 7-4 shows the basic elements of a range ambiguity artifact for pulsed Doppler.

These deeper reflections can enter the system only if they come from particular ranges. Specifically, echoes can effectively enter the range gate only when they come from exact multiples of the gated range. For example, if the range gate position is 10 cm, then signals coming from 20 cm could also reach the transducer at the same time. These signals return later than the original transmit-receive cycle.

It is these late-arriving, deeper echo signals that produce the ambiguity artifact. Later, we will use this "temporal resonance" in a special application of pulsed Doppler to increase the maximum Doppler shift frequency limit.

Connecting Echo-Signal Phase and Direction

For our purpose here, phase and time are nearly synonymous terms. In addition, changes in phase are equivalent to a frequency. We can express phase as time within a signal cycle, and this time is expressed in units of degrees. A complete cycle contains 360°; a phase shift of 90° represents one quarter of a cycle. Thus, a signal shifted 90° is moved in time one quarter of a cycle.

A phase shift can be positive or negative. For our discussion, a negative phase

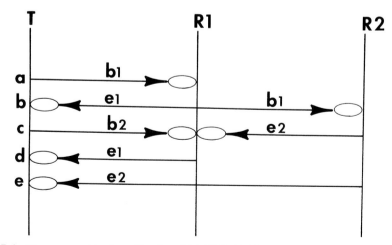

Figure 7-4   The range ambiguity artifact from high PRFs. In this case, signals from range 2 (*R2*) can enter the system because they arrive at the same time as echoes from range 1 (*R1*). *a,* The first burst (*b1*) leaves the transducer face (*T*) and reaches the depth *R1*. *b,* Echo *e1* returns to the transducer while burst *b1* continues and reaches *R2*. *c,* On the next cycle, burst 2 (*b2*), reaches *R1* as the echo 2 (*e2*) reaches *R1*. *d* and *e,* Now *e1* and *e2* arrive at the transducer at the same time, superimposed.

shift for a signal means that it arrives earlier, and therefore a cycle would start earlier than normal. A positive phase shift, on the other hand, means that the signal arrives later in time, and therefore a cycle would start later than normal. These time relationships are shown in Figure 7-5. We can compare two signals for phase, however, and describe their relationship using the words *leading* and *lagging*. In this instance, one signal can lead or lag another in phase (time).

In Chapter 6, we learned about the basic role of the quadrature phase detector in detecting motion and separating it into direction. Let's examine in more detail how phase measurements can show motion and direction.

The quadrature phase detector uses the phase or timing between a master oscillator and a returning echo signal to detect motion and determine its direction. An echo source moving toward the transducer increases the echo signal frequency, causing the echo signal to lead the master oscillator signal. Moving away from the transducer lowers the echo signal frequency. This, in turn, makes the echo signal lag the master oscillator signal.

By combining the input echo signal with an in-phase and out-of-phase master oscillator signal, two new signals appear at the output of the circuit (Fig. 7-6). One output channel is the inphase or I channel, and the other is the quadrature or Q channel. The I channel can be thought of as the forward channel, the Q channel as the reverse channel. These are functional labels rather than electronic separations. In fact, when motion occurs toward the transducer, the I channel leads the Q channel by 90°. When motion occurs away from the transducer, the Q channel leads the I channel by 90°. This 90° phase shift gives this detector its "quadrature" label, which means 90° phase shift.

A CW system can detect motion by sampling the frequency change directly. This measurement comes from comparing the frequency of a returning echo signal with that of the master oscillator. Although this permits a measure of the frequency change, information about the direction of motion vanishes in this detection process.[4] Moving toward or away from the transducer produces either a positive or negative frequency difference, respectively. But because a negative frequency has no physical reality, equal speeds toward or away from the transducer produce the same result.

A way to manage this problem is to mix the Doppler shift frequency with yet another frequency. The second frequency is higher than the largest expected Doppler shift frequency in the system. This technique is shown in Figure 7-7. By adding an offset frequency to the Doppler shift frequency (heterodyning), a new signal results that can show both the direction of motion and the speed.[5] Now, moving away from the transducer lowers the new signal frequency, and moving toward the transducer increases this frequency.

Another way of detecting the phase and frequency changes associated with the Doppler effect is an autocorrelator circuit.[6] This circuit tests successive echo signals

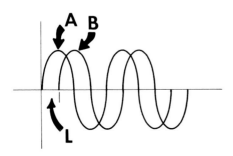

Figure 7-5 Phase or timing relationships between signals. Signals *A* and *B* do not have the same time base. In this case, *A* can be seen to lead (*L*) signal *B*, or signal *B* can be thought to lag behind *A*. Choosing the reference defines leading or lagging.

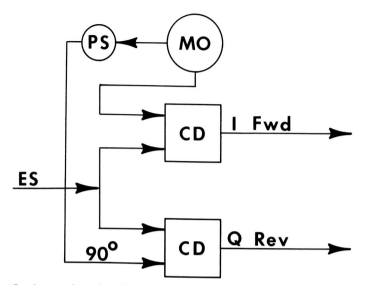

Figure 7-6   Quadrature phase detection. In this detection scheme, the master oscillator (*MO*) reference signal proceeds to a pair of coherent detectors (*CD*). One signal is inphase and the other signal is phase shifted (*PS*) 90°. The inphase and out-of-phase signals enter the detectors at the same time as the echo signal (*ES*). The two outputs, *I* and *Q*, are then out of phase. The inphase (*I*) channel leads the quadrature (*Q*) channel by 90° with forward motion, and lags it by 90° with reversed motion.

against one another for changes in phase and frequency. Movement toward the transducer, for example, will cause successive echo signals to lead the previous echo signals. Movement away from the transducer will cause successive echo signals to lag the previous echo signals. This system requires either a signal storage scheme or a time delay circuit to hold the first signal through a delay period of one pulse-listen cycle. The organization for this scheme is shown in Figure 7-8.

Chapter 6 introduced the phaser diagram to show the phase-dependent events in Doppler ultrasound. This diagram also gives a good graphic representation of the major signal separation problem in Doppler ultrasound. This separation is especially difficult in the CW Doppler system, because so much of the beam intercepts stationary tissue.

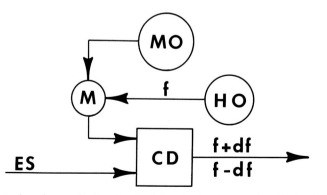

Figure 7-7   Detecting changes in direction by heterodyning frequencies. Motion information can come from the echo signal (*ES*) by mixing (*M*) the master oscillator (*MO*) signals with an offset frequency (*f*) from a heterodyne oscillator (*HO*). The new signal is coherently detected (*CD*) to produce Doppler frequencies above (*f* + *df*) and below (*f* − *df*) the reference frequency (*f*) set by the heterodyne oscillator.

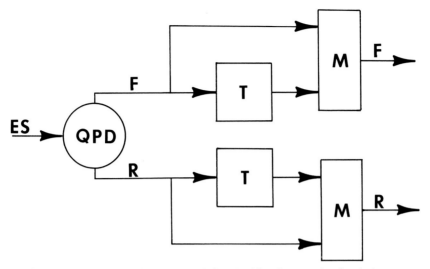

Figure 7-8   Detecting motion using autocorrelation. In this scheme, echo signals from successive pulse-listen cycles are compared in a demodulator (*M*). The time delay (*T*) holds the previous signal for comparison with the succeeding signals. In this diagram, *ES* is the echo signal, *QPD* is the quadrature phase detector, *F* and *R* are inphase and quadrature channels that become forward and reverse signal channels.

Such tissue produces very large, steady signals that do not change in phase. In contrast, the moving segments of tissue and RBCs produce very small signals that not only vary in phase, but also in amplitude. They show up on the phaser diagram as a vector rotating about the tip of the large tissue signal (Fig. 7-9).

To put things in proper scale, the RBCs produce echo signals that can be 40 to 60 dB *below* the tissue signal amplitudes. This represents a 100:1 to 1,000:1 ratio in amplitude. Even under the best conditions, flow information could have an amplitude only 1% of that of the tissue leakage signal. By limiting signals to just blood (the sample volume is confined to a vessel lumen), a pulsed Doppler system markedly reduces the signal separation problem.

Detecting the Doppler Shift Frequency

Sometimes, changing our point of view about a particular process can lead to new understanding. One such new view is to look at the Doppler effect as a process that modulates or changes a carrier signal.[7] Just as audio signals in a radio studio shift the carrier frequency (FM) of a radio transmitter, the Doppler effect shifts the frequency of an ultrasonic echo. From this perspective, echo-source motion modulates the reflecting ultrasound, and the signal that returns is a carrier frequency, shifted because of the Doppler effect. The Doppler shift signal, then, becomes a "sideband." Thus, the Doppler shift frequency can be separated out using single sideband-detecting techniques from radio communications.

The quadrature phase detector and some of the sideband-filtering techniques used in Doppler ultrasound come directly from radio engineering.[8] Indeed, quadrature phase detection depends upon the equivalence of frequency and changing phase. It is this equivalence that also makes the echo signal rotate about its center in the phaser diagram.

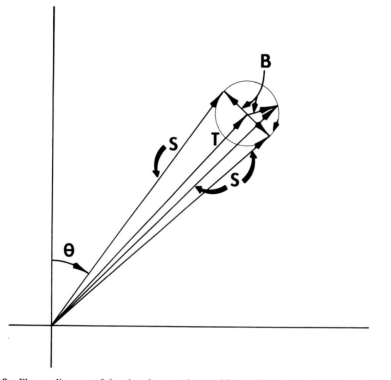

Figure 7-9   Phaser diagram of the signal separation problem in Doppler. In general, tissue signals (*T*) are much larger than blood signals (*B*). Furthermore, the blood signals are changing in phase (θ) because of motion. The blood and tissue signals add to form the vector result (*S*), which changes phase as the blood signal changes. The signal processing problem is to separate *B* from *T*.

This notion of phase detection also makes sense because it is difficult to measure the very small changes in frequency that occur in the small sampling intervals typical of pulsed-Doppler systems. Although the frequency of a returning echo may change little, the equivalent change in phase can be much larger. In addition, phase-sensing circuits can be very sensitive. The Doppler shift frequency emerges from the sampling that occurs with each pulse-listen cycle. The final output frequency takes shape from the many samples that occur each second (PRF). As a result, the PRF plays a central role in accurately estimating the Doppler shift frequency.

If the changes in phase are too large between sampling intervals, a process called high-frequency aliasing occurs. This problem and some of its solutions are detailed in Chapter 8.

Sometimes a connection between ideas appears so complete and elegant that it is worth examining, even though it may contribute little to running a sonograph. Its value lies in creating understanding. One such connection is the derivation of the Doppler equation by considering only the changes in phase associated with the echo-ranging process.

Consider first a transmitted burst of ultrasound that has a 0° phase angle at time zero. Because phase is expressed in degrees, a phase angle is an appropriate expression to use. At some distance, *d,* an echo starts returning to the transducer. When the echo arrives, it will have a phase angle, P, determined by the frequency of the ultrasound, F_0, and the round trip time of flight, T_d. The equation is

$$P = F_0 T_d \tag{7.1}$$

The transmitted frequency, F_0, is a constant for the system; thus, any change in P is a function of the time of flight, T_d, only. If we take a time derivative to express this rate of change, the equation becomes

$$dP/dt = F_0 (dT_d/dt) \tag{7.2}$$

T_d, however, can be restated as the target range, Z, and the velocity of propagation, c. This equation is

$$T_d = 2 (Z/c). \tag{7.3}$$

In turn, the time derivative of the time of flight, based on Equation 7.3 is

$$dT_d/dt = (2/c)(dZ/dt) \tag{7.4}$$

where dZ/dt is really the echo-source closing velocity, V. Equation 7.4 becomes

$$dT_d/dt = 2 V/c \tag{7.5}$$

Substituting Equation 6.5 back into Equation 6.2, we get

$$dP/dt = 2 F_0 V/c \tag{7.6}$$

A frequency is, of course, a change in phase, giving

$$dP/dt = Df = 2 F_0 (V/c) \tag{7.7}$$

where Df is the Doppler shift frequency, and V is the closing velocity between the ultrasound source and the echo source. Equation 7.7 is the Doppler equation, derived from the phase changes associated with a moving target in an echo-ranging system. Thus, the process of reconstructing the Doppler shift frequency by sampling phase changes is a real connection.

Analyzing Doppler Shift Frequencies

Except for the most simple and unreal situations, the Doppler shift frequency signal is not a simple, single tone. The detected Doppler signal is always a mix of many signals from many different echo sources moving through the ultrasound beam at the same time. The actual signal is the superposition of many smaller signals, added in a simple manner. Extracting these component frequencies is possible because the individual contributing signals continue to exist within the complex signal.

Although we speak of the "Fourier components" of a signal mix, not all methods of isolating these frequency components are Fourier analysis. And if the extraction is not based on Fourier analysis, these new frequency components are not truly Fourier components.[9] Fourier frequency components, however, do have a special characteristic: they are mathematically orthogonal, i.e., the components are independent of one another and are not functions of any other components.[10] Because other methods of frequency separation beyond Fourier analysis seek these same independent frequencies, the analytical results are nearly the same. The sameness of these component frequencies, regardless of analytical approach, demonstrates an unexpected connection between the mathematics of Fourier and the physical world.

Exploring the various methods for extracting the fundamental frequency components of a signal mix not only provides additional insight into the problems of deciphering complex signals, but also illustrates the limitations of some of these techniques.

Multifilter Analysis

One of the very first methods for isolating the frequency components within a complicated Doppler shift signal was multifilter analysis.[5] In this technique, a number of filters, each tuned to different frequencies, operate on the complex signal to separate out the components of the Doppler shift signal (Fig. 7-10). The accuracy of this separation depends upon the number of filters used and how narrow their bandwidths are.

Multifilter analysis is a brute-force method of obtaining frequency components. And unless the filters have very narrow bandwidths (i.e., tuned to very specific frequencies), the derived frequency components may not really be Fourier components. This difference comes from the lack of orthogonal qualities in a multifilter system. As a result, the frequency separation may not be as good as a pure mathematical analysis. Filters are seldom so frequency specific that frequencies close but not equal to the central filter frequency cannot influence the filter function. Thus, the frequency components may not all be entirely independent.

Early use of multifilter analysis was hampered by poor filter design and a non-real-time function.[11] The early analyzers used voice analysis filters or more complicated, electronically controlled filters that could change frequency. The Doppler shift signal under investigation was transferred to tape and formed into a continuous loop. Then the signal being analyzed was played repeatedly as new filters were switched in or an electronically controlled filter changed frequency. The results appeared on a circulating strip chart, with each replay of the signal slowly building the final spectral analysis.

These systems were difficult to use because the filters were analog and passive,

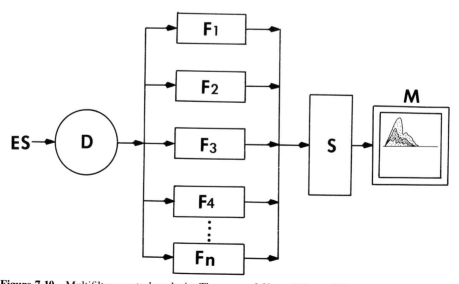

Figure 7-10 Multifilter spectral analysis. The array of filters (*F1* . . . *Fn*) are chosen to provide a frequency separation that approximates Fourier frequency components. The echo signal (*ES*) is Doppler detected (*D*) and the complex composite signals passes through the filters. The output is summed (*S*) for display and finally appears on a monitor (*M*).

requiring many components that had to be stable over time and different frequencies. Because the filter was a passive circuit, it reduced the signal amplitudes. And because the display used a gray scale to depict frequency component amplitudes, each of the filter channels had to have a similar gain and bandwidth. In general, this was not a clinically valuable approach, although the results from these early experiments provided information on what to expect in the Doppler signal spectrum.

Newer techniques use integrated circuits to gang together active filters. These new filter designs have two major advantages: first, they can provide real-time analysis of the signals; and second, they are very much alike in gain and bandwidth. As a result, the frequency components derived with such a filter system are usually much closer to those determined by Fourier analysis.

The Zero Crossing Detector

Probably the most widely used of early forms of frequency analysis was the zero-crossing detector (ZCD).[12] First thought to be a quantitative tool, the ZCD seemed to have an output useful for determining mean values, which would reveal volume flow through various vascular compartments.[13] The results were disappointing, however. Nevertheless, the ZCD produced much of the early information about the behavior of blood flow in the vascular system, and it provided a good qualitative look at vascular events.

The ZCD uses the basic property of any sinusoidal function: it crosses zero at a rate proportional to the sinusoidal frequency. Increasing the signal frequency, for example, shortens the time interval between crossings (Fig. 7-11). The ZCD circuit puts out a pulse with constant amplitude and width for each zero crossing. The interval between these pulses is proportional to the frequency of the input signal. And, of course, the reciprocal to these intervals is equivalent to frequency, just as the frequency of a wave is equal to the reciprocal of its period.

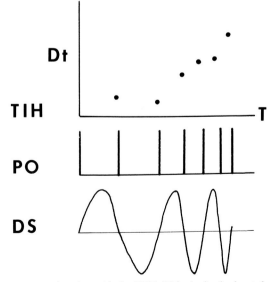

Figure 7-11 Frequency approximation with the ZCD. This device looks at the zero crossings in the Doppler signal (*DS*), producing a pulse output (PO) for each crossing. The interval between pulses is inversely related to frequency, and appears as a dot on the time interval histogram (*TIH*). Here the X-axis is time (*t*) and the Y-axis is the inverse of the time interval between pulses (*Dt*).

The output from the ZCD then enters a circuit that converts the pulse interval information into frequency. In the ZCD display, the interval frequency appears on the Y-axis of a graph, and time appears on the X-axis. The result is the time interval histogram, the display format for Doppler systems using a ZCD.

At first, the ZCD appeared to be a quantitative tool because of its response during laboratory measurements. Putting a signal into a ZCD and plotting the results with changing frequency produced correlations between input and output signals of greater than 98%.[14] Clearly, the ZCD was able to quantitate frequencies in a Doppler shift signal.

Correlations in the field, however, were very disappointing: the ZCD did not show good quantitation at all. Meanwhile, back in the engineering lab, frequency input-output correlations were still high. Something was different about typical Doppler shift signals that prevented the ZCD from handling them.

The answer was signal complexity. In the laboratory, single frequencies are used to measure the response of a ZCD, and in this simple situation, the ZCD responds well. Real Doppler shift signals, however, are very complex with many of the frequency components modulating the signal but not crossing zero. As a result, the ZCD has a bias toward the low-frequency, high-amplitude components of a signal mix, as shown in Figure 7-12. This sort of inherent signal weighting prevents the ZCD from becoming a truly quantitative device.

In addition to signal weighting, the ZCD is also unable to separate a signal crossing zero from a noise spike crossing zero. Because of this zero-crossing "blindness," the ZCD is very sensitive to the presence of noise and requires a good signal-to-noise ratio to work best.

The ZCD is still used in some systems as a means of examining the qualitative

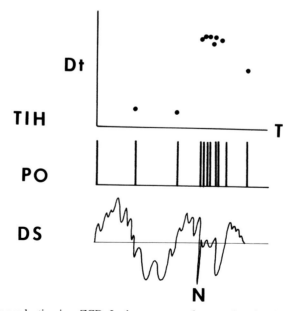

Figure 7-12   Error production in a ZCD. In the presence of a complex signal mix (*DS*), the ZCD confuses noise (*N*) and high-frequency components. Furthermore, the high-frequency components on the waveform are invisible to the detector, except close to the zero line. *PO* is the pulse output, *TIH* is the time interval histogram, *T* is time, and *Dt* is the estimated frequency.

aspects of a Doppler signal. The quantitation mantle has now fallen on the shoulders of the next technology in line, the fast Fourier transform system. Nevertheless, much of the early information about blood flow came from the ZCD. These data are still useful today, provided we keep the limitations of the ZCD in mind.

The Fast Fourier Transform Device

The word "fast" in the title of this section really suggests that a "slow" Fourier transform exists, and it does. Fourier analysis was first a mathematical technique that separated complex, periodic wave forms into simple, sinusoidal components.[9] Such an analysis could be complete but hardly fast. Then, in the 1960s, an algorithm to compute the complex Fourier series appeared that made the analysis available to the computer.[5] This algorithm was the fast Fourier transform or FFT. Other operators besides Fourier transforms are available,[10] but they do not handle the wide range of functions possible with an FFT.

Along with an ability to handle a greater number of functions, the output of an FFT analysis consists of individual frequency components that are mathematically "orthogonal." That means the components are not functions of one another, and therefore, they do not interact. As a result, frequency estimates are more accurate and cleaner than with the ZCD.

At the heart of the FFT process is the assumption that any complicated waveform consists of a simple summation of sine waves that vary in amplitude, phase, and frequency. In addition, these component waves do not lose identity when they add, and they emerge out of hiding, so to speak, by applying the correct operator. In this case, the operator is the Fourier frequency analysis technique.

The output from an FFT device consists of individual frequency components, expressed as amplitudes and frequencies. The phase information is not essential to ultrasound applications and disappears in the extraction.

The frequency analysis depends upon a digital computer system to extract the information. The basic steps for an FFT device are shown in Figure 7-13. Because the

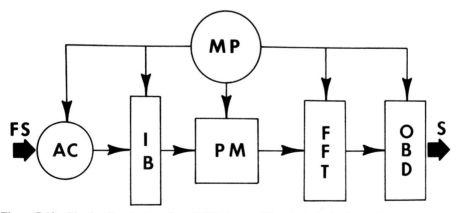

Figure 7-13   The fast Fourier transform (*FFT*) device. The whole device is run by the master processor (*MP*), typically a microprocessor. The frequency containing signal (*FS*) enters through an analog-to-digital converter (*AC*), and these binary numbers are stored in an input buffer (*IB*). The numbers then go to the processor memory (*PM*) and finally to the algorithm (*FFT*). The output signals from the FFT functions go to an output buffer and display circuit (*OBD*), and finally appear as frequency component signals (*S*).

analysis is digital, the output frequencies are not continuous, but discrete, and appear as a digital image pixel (Fig. 7-14). The Y-axis of this pixel represents a range of frequencies called a frequency bin. The X-axis of the pixel is time, representing the FFT sampling period. Typical time values for medical applications of an FFT system range from 5–10 ms to as long as 300 ms. In addition, each pixel has a gray scale intensity that represents the component frequency amplitude.

Under the right conditions, the intensity of the frequency component is proportional to the number of RBCs traveling together at the same velocity and time. The pixels in the display also show the range of frequencies, which represents the range of RBC velocities. In this manner, the Doppler display has a strong link to the physical events in the vascular compartment.

Doppler frequency analysis using an FFT device requires a computer or its equivalent to calculate the Fourier frequency components. The output from the Doppler detector, however, is an analog signal, so one of the early steps in FFT analysis is to convert the analog signal to a digital signal. An analog-to-digital converter or ADC makes this conversion (Fig. 7-13). In addition, only a small portion of the Doppler signal can be processed at any time, and that requires sampling the Doppler signal for a finite period. These sampling intervals are in the order of 5–10 ms.

The ADC converts the analog signal into a sequence of binary numbers that represent the changing analog signal amplitude during the sampling period. The accuracy of this conversion depends on the number of bits used to describe a number in the ADC. For example, if the ADC uses only 4 bits to define values, then only 16 values are possible. Alternately, 5 bits permits 32 values. If the ADC is to depict accurately the small changes in the analog signal shape that represent higher frequencies, then the digital samplings must be rather small. Good ADCs for FFT applications often use 10-bit or 12-bit words.

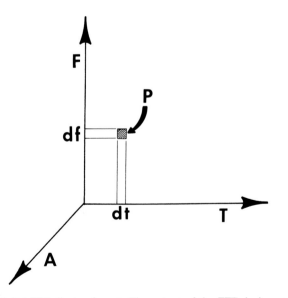

Figure 7-14   The digital FFT display format. The output of the FFT device appears as a digital spectrum, with frequency components (*F*) on the Y-axis, time (*T*) on the X-axis, and amplitude (*A*) of the components in gray scale intensity (Z-axis). The sampling time for the FFT is *dt*, and the range of frequencies treated alike or as a frequency bin is *df*. *P* is the individual picture element (pixel).

Out of the ADC comes a series of binary numbers that go through a buffer before being "number crunched" by the computer and FFT algorithm (Fig. 7-13). The buffer is a memory used to store the signal temporarily to keep events correctly timed in the digital system. After the component frequency outputs are stored in a buffer, they go through a digital-to-analog converter (DAC). This converter carries out two functions: first, it changes the digital output of the computer into signals capable of display; second, an assignment between the digital values and display format voltages occurs. If the display is a gray-scale image, then the assignment works much like postprocessing in a digital scan converter. The processing assigns a gray scale value to the digital numbers coming from the FFT circuit. If the image depicts frequency components in color, then the output signals are converted to a color with the characteristics of hue (wave length), saturation (purity), and intensity (brightness).

In general, an inverse relationship exists between the sampling interval and the number of frequency components that an FFT device can calculate. As the sampling interval increases, the frequency bins can become smaller. For example, if a 10-ms sampling interval divides its frequency range into 128 frequency intervals or bins, a 5-ms sampling may only do half as well, with 64 bins. Choosing the right sampling interval, then, depends in part on the accuracy needs of the Fourier component analysis. In general, the longer the sampling interval, the greater the accuracy of the FFT analysis.[5]

Digitally sampling an analog signal sets a limit to the highest frequency the sampling can accurately depict. This highest frequency is called the Nyquist limit. The Nyquist limit is either the sampling frequency divided by two, or in some FFT systems, equal to the sampling frequency itself.[15] For an FFT device sampling at 10-ms intervals, the ADC sampling rate determines this limit, which may be greater than 1 MHz. As a result, no practical upper limit exists for Doppler signal analysis with an FFT system because the Doppler shift signals are within the audio spectrum and well below the radio frequency sampling rate of the FFT device.

Such an open upper limit is ideal for a CW Doppler system, which also has no practical upper limit on the Doppler shift frequencies it can handle. The pulsed Doppler system, however, does not have this limitless quality. A pulsed-Doppler system is effectively sampling the Doppler shift frequency at the PRF. This places the Nyquist limit for most ultrasound systems at PRF divided by two, because the PRF is much lower than the FFT sampling frequency at the ADC. With some systems, this limit can become the PRF if the signal processing uses complex mathematics (real and imaginary numbers).[16]

The existence of a maximum frequency limit suggests a lower limit as well. The sampling duration of the FFT device sets the lower limit.[16] The lowest frequency is the smallest number of whole cycles that can fit within the sampling duration, typically one cycle. A 10-ms interval, then, could not contain a signal lower than 100 Hz, which has a period of 10 ms.

The impact of the FFT device on Doppler signal analysis is reminiscent of that caused by the introduction of the digital scan converter to B-mode imaging. Moving from the analog to the digital domain introduces a new set of desirable parameters to Doppler signal processing. For example, the FFT system performs a more stable analysis of the Doppler shift frequencies than earlier analytical designs, all on a real-time format. FFT analysis can quantify the Doppler signal component frequencies and amplitudes with an accuracy hard to achieve otherwise. The FFT system lacks the inherent biases of the ZCD, and provides discrete component values unavailable to the latter system. And finally, FFT digital data is accessible by outside computers for additional, advanced analysis. Modern FFT analysis has clearly provided a set of unequaled benefits to the clinical user.

Complex Numbers and the FFT   One of the more subtle mathematical manipulations of the FFT algorithm is the use of complex numbers. In this case, complex does not mean complicated. Instead, it means a set of numbers with unusual mathematical properties.

Complex mathematics came about because some equations exist that require special solutions. For example, let's consider the equation

$$x^2 + 3 = 0$$
$$x^2 = -3$$
$$x = \sqrt{-3} \text{ or}$$
$$x = (\sqrt{-1})(\sqrt{3})$$

Taking the square root of -1 is not possible within the real number system, and thus, it is said to be an imaginary number.[9]

Complex numbers have the form that, given any two numbers, a and b, then a complex number $a + ib$ exists, where i is the $\sqrt{-1}$. The complex number, then, has two parts, a real part, expressed by a, and an imaginary part expressed by ib.

Although this seems a bit unconnected with the signals that come out of an FFT device, a subtle and valuable connection exists. Using complex numbers to calculate Fourier components yields a very agreeable result.

To understand the potential benefits of complex mathematics in calculating Fourier components, we need to look at sampling and signal conversion. In a sonograph, sampling occurs at an ADC. We also need to look at the signals in terms of frequency rather than time.

Converting an analog signal to a digital signal starts with sampling. This conversion centers on a sample-and-hold function. In this function, a circuit samples the incoming analog signal at some time and holds that value until the next sample. The circuit output carries the sampled value for a short time and then returns to its baseline value, zero. The continuous analog signal now becomes a set of very narrow signals of equal duration, but changing in height (value) with each sampling. These very narrow samplings rise and fall steeply, creating a wide range of Fourier frequencies within each sample.

Thus, sampling a signal for later digital processing creates a very wide spectrum of positive and negative frequencies. These frequencies center on the harmonics of the *sampling* frequency, as shown in Figure 7-15. Normally, we have no use for these higher ordered harmonics, so they vanish as the signal stream passes through a low-pass filter.

The low-pass filtering leaves only a band of frequencies spread over a width equal to the sampling frequency. If frequency components within the sampled signal exceed the bandwidth of the low-pass filter, high-frequency aliasing occurs. Aliasing is an engineering term that means the high frequencies begin to look like lower frequencies. On a spectral display, aliasing looks as if the original signal is wrapping around the display. For example, as the high frequencies in a spectrum exceed the aliasing limit, they appear as lower frequencies in the opposite directional channel. Figure 7-16 shows this wrap-around process.

Sampling a real value signal produces a set of positive and negative frequencies that are symmetrical about the zero signal value. This relationship is depicted in Figure 7-17, which shows the positive and negative frequencies mirrored about the zero line.

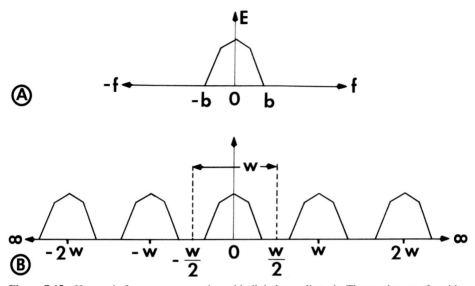

Figure 7-15 Harmonic frequency generation with digital sampling. **A,** The starting set of positive and negative analog frequencies (*f*) as a function of energy (*E*); *b* represents the positive and negative frequency boundaries of the spectrum. **B,** Digital sampling generates a host of spectrums, each centered on a harmonic (*w, 2w, 3w,* etc.) of the sampling frequency (*w*). These spectra theoretically proceed to infinity in both directions. Low pass filtering removes these high-frequency components.

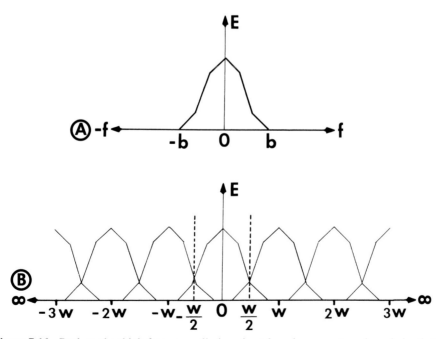

Figure 7-16 Real number high-frequency aliasing. **A,** +*b,* −*b* are spectrum boundaries that are larger than the sampling bandwidth that create high frequency "wings," **B,** that overlap into the next sampling interval. This makes the high frequencies appear as low frequencies in the opposite direction. *E* is the frequency component energy, and *w* is the sampling frequency.

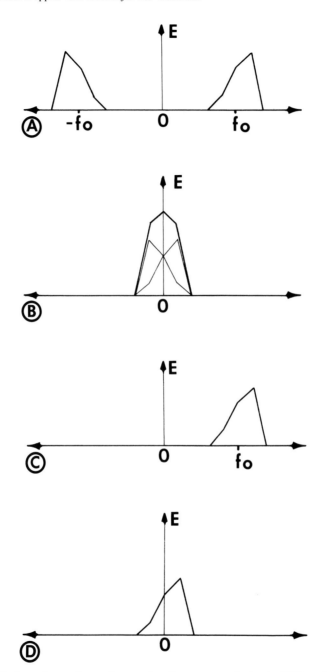

Figure 7-17   Real number and complex number frequency analysis. **A,** FFT analysis of a real number produces both positive and negative frequencies of the spectrum, centered on $+fo$ and $-fo$. **B,** When these spectra are detected, they transfer to the base band and superimpose on one another at the zero frequency. As a result, only half the sampling bandwidth can be used without high-frequency aliasing. In a pulsed Doppler system, this is PRF/2. **C,** FFT of a complex number produces a single asymmetric spectrum centered on fo. **D,** When this spectrum is detected and appears at the zero frequency, only one spectrum appears, and the whole sampling bandwidth is available without aliasing. Now the pulsed Doppler aliasing frequency becomes PRF. E is the frequency component energy; fo is the spectrum center frequency.

When we remove absolute frequencies and consider only changes in frequency (detection), the two spectra overlay one another. Because of the mirror symmetry, only half the sampling bandwidth is useful. Aliasing occurs, then, when the highest frequency exceeds the bandwidth divided by two. The bandwidth, of course, is equal to the sampling frequency. And this is the connection to a typical Doppler system. Thus, aliasing occurs in a typical pulsed Doppler system when the highest Doppler shift frequency (the signal being sampled at PRF) exceeds PRF divided by two.

Sampling a signal with both real and imaginary parts (mathematically complex) produces a single set of frequencies that are *not* symmetrical to the zero frequency line (Figure 7-17, C and D). The nonsymmetrical set of frequencies permits full use of the sampling bandwidth. If frequencies do exceed the bandwidth in either direction, moving the filtering bandwidth will include the higher frequencies. Thus, the maximum aliasing frequency turns out not to be sampling frequency divided by two, but the sampling frequency itself.

This simple mathematical effect doubles the useful range of the sampling process. In a pulsed-Doppler system, then, using complex signals for processing extends the effective aliasing limit to PRF and not PRF divided by two. It is a subtle effect with a real clinical benefit.

A system that aliases at PRF permits a higher Doppler carrier frequency without aliasing. A higher carrier frequency means that lower blood velocities that were formerly invisible become visible. In other words, the Doppler system can handle a wider range of blood velocities that appear in both arterial and venous disease.

References

1. Havlice, JF, and Taenzer, JC. Medical ultrasonic imaging: An overview of principles and instrumentation. *Proc IEEE* 67:620–641, 1979.
2. Baker, DW, Forster, FK, and Daigle, RE. Doppler Principles and Techniques. *In* Fry, FJ (ed): *Ultrasound: Its Applications in Medicine and Biology,* Part 1. New York: Elsevier Scientific, 1978, pp 161–287.
3. Goldstein, A. Range ambiguities in real-time ultrasound. *J Clin Ultrasound* 9:83–90, 1981.
4. Waxham, RD. Doppler ultrasound. *Radiology Today,* April/May 1980.
5. Atkinson, P, Woodcock, JP. *Doppler Ultrasound and Its Use in Clinical Measurement.* New York: Academic Press, 1982, pp 63, 101, 110.
6. Omoto, R (ed). *Color Atlas of Real-Time Two-Dimensional Doppler Echocardiology.* Tokyo: Shidan-To-Chiryo, 1984, p 10.
7. Wells, PNT. *Physical Principles of Ultrasonic Diagnosis.* New York: Academic Press, 1969, p 200.
8. McLeod, FD. A directional Doppler flowmeter. *Digest 7th International Congress for Medical and Biological Engineering,* p 271, 1967.
9. Kreyszig, E. *Advanced Engineering Mathematics.* New York: John Wiley, 1962, pp 464–491.
10. Davis, HF. *Fourier Series and Orthogonal Functions.* Boston: Allyn and Bacon, 1963, p 30.
11. Johnston, KW, Maruzzo, BC, Kassam, M., et al. Methods for obtaining, processing and quantifying Doppler blood velocity waveforms. *In* Nicolaides, AN and Yao, JST (eds): *Investigation of Vascular Disorders.* New York: Churchill Livingston. 1981, pp 532–558.
12. Lorch, G, Rubenstein, S, Baker, D, et al. Doppler echocardiography use of a graphical display. *Circulation* 56:576–585, 1977.
13. Gill, RW. Performance of the mean frequency Doppler modulator. *Ultrasound Med Biol* 5:237–247, 1979.

14. Hoeks, APG, Peeters, HHPM, Ruissen, CJ, et al. A novel frequency estimator for sampled Doppler signals. *IEEE Trans Biomed Eng* BME-31:212–220, 1985.
15. Ramirez, RW. *The FFT: Fundamentals and Concepts.* Beaverton, OR: Tektronix, Inc., 1975, pp 4–36.
16. Hatle, L and Angelsen, B. *Doppler Ultrasound in Cardiology.* Philadelphia: Lea & Febiger, 1982, pp 205, 211.

8

Duplex Imaging and
Other Advanced Techniques

Although the first paper on duplex imaging appeared in 1974,[1] only now are these devices gaining widespread popularity. The original design grew out of a fundamental problem that continues to plague the examination of vessels with Doppler. Continuous wave (CW) and pulsed Doppler offer no unique spatial information about which vessel out of many might be the Doppler signal source. To diminish this uncertainty, duplex systems bring together a real-time, B-mode imaging system and a Doppler signal processor into a single, integrated machine. The image provides a look at the vascular anatomy, while the Doppler system provides information about flow events within the vessel.

The first duplex system used pulsed Doppler, but many current designs offer both pulsed and CW Doppler in the same device. The real-time images can come from linear arrays, mechanical sector scanners, or phased arrays. Despite these differences, duplex systems still separate into two major groups, based on how imaging and Doppler processing share time. There are true duplex systems and time-share duplex systems. The former can also be simple or advanced.

First True Duplex System

By definition, a duplex system is one that combines imaging and Doppler processing into a single, integrated machine (Fig. 8-1). The image contains both a B-mode, gray-scale image and a Doppler spectrum. Further refining this notion, a true duplex system is one that uses the same signal to obtain imaging and Doppler information.

This organization means that the same signal provides both the echo-signal amplitude to produce an image and the echo-signal phase and frequency to extract Doppler information. These signal-processing steps are not only parallel but often happen at the same time within the machine. They are finally brought together into a single integrated image. A more accurate description of this simultaneous processing for amplitude and Doppler data is synchronous signal processing. The first true duplex system was the M/Q system,[2] a combination of M-mode and pulsed-Doppler functions.

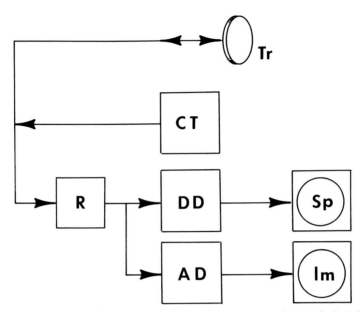

Figure 8-1   A true duplex system. The organization uses a common receiver (R) for both image (AD) and Doppler (DD) detection. CT is a coherent transmitter, Tr is the transducer, Sp is the spectral display, and Im is the gray-scale image display.

A time-share duplex system seeks the same information, but interweaves the Doppler and imaging functions. The system collects data sequentially, first some image information, then some Doppler information, and again image information. This separation in events is so strong, it uses different echo signals for each function, as shown in Figure 8-2. By interweaving the different events properly, a time-share duplex system can provide an updating image and a Doppler spectral output to the display at the same time, even though the data are not gathered simultaneously. Hence, this is an asynchronous signal-processing system.

Because image and Doppler signal processing in a true duplex system are simultaneous, it uses the same transducer for both Doppler and imaging. The shape, phase, and frequency content of the transmitted burst are central to this signal processing.

For example, the burst must be short for good axial resolution but long enough for a good Doppler signal-to-noise ratio. To satisfy both needs, the transmitter voltage is usually a sine wave with a known phase and frequency. Good imaging requires a short, sharp electrical pulse into a heavily damped transducer, producing a wide range of frequencies. In contrast, Doppler processing needs a lightly damped transducer, producing a narrow range of frequencies. The right compromises in design will give a transducer acceptable behavior for both imaging and Doppler.

The M/Q Organization

M/Q is a combination of two elements: an M-mode display (hence the *M*), and a display of flow events using a Doppler spectrum (hence the Q, a mathematical symbol often used to represent flow). The M-mode display is a particularly useful way of looking at motion within the heart. Before real-time B-mode imaging, M-mode stand-alone systems were already heavily used in echocardiography.

An M-mode display comes from a moving B-mode trace. The echo signals return-

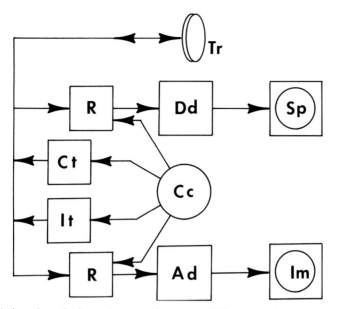

Figure 8-2 A time-share duplex system. In this system, different signals are processed for image and Doppler information, despite a common transducer, *Tr*. *Ct* is the Doppler coherent transmitter; the incoherent image transmitter is *It*. Each channel has separate receivers (*R*), and separate detection. *Dd* is the Doppler detector; *Ad* is the amplitude detector. The displays are *Sp* for Doppler spectrum, and *Im* for gray-scale image. *Cc* is the common clock for coordinating events in the machine.

ing from cardiac structures are converted into a gray-scale dots, with an intensity proportional to the echo-signal amplitude. Moving these dots across the screen at a steady rate shows how the interfaces are moving. With this display, it is easy to identify major cardiac structures and to follow both fast and slow motion over the cardiac cycle. Combining motion characteristics with major landmarks, an M/Q system can accurately site a Doppler sample volume in specific cardiac chambers and flow channels.

The M/Q system is a true duplex (synchronous) system, and uses a common transducer and transmitter (Fig. 8-3). A gated transmitter delivers several cycles of driving voltage at the Doppler operating frequency. This sets the ultrasound burst length and amplitude. On the receiver side, the system processes the returning echo signals into a B-mode trace. It moves across the screen to form an M-mode display (Fig. 8-3).

To satisfy Doppler signal processing needs, the ultrasound transmitting burst may be a little longer than that typically used for imaging. Some current ultrasound receivers may be sensitive enough to do away with this requirement, however. The additional burst length can degrade the imaging axial resolution. As a result, many early systems had a broad, flat M-mode trace because of the long transmitting burst.

Within an M/Q system, the transducer changes an arriving echo into an echo signal. It then amplifies the signal, while at the same time reducing the incoming signal dynamic range with time gain compensation.

The signal path next divides into two pathways. The imaging signal path leads to a conventional amplitude detector. At the same time, the Doppler signal path leads to a quadrature phase detector (QPD). This detector uses phase changes to ascertain motion and separate the Doppler signal path into forward and reverse channels. These channels represent motion toward and away from the transducer.

The M-mode display provides a single line of sight through an organ of interest

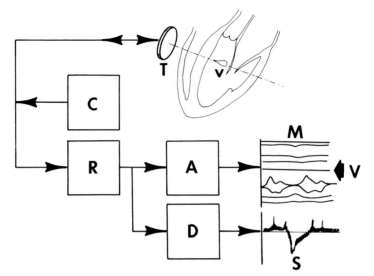

Figure 8-3   Organization of an M/Q duplex system. This system employs an M-mode display (*M*) and spectrum (*S*) for Doppler information. *T* is the transducer, *v* is the sample volume location in the cardiac anatomy, *C* is the coherent transmitter, *R* is the receiver, *A* and *D* are amplitude and Doppler detection, respectively, and *V* is the sample volume and receiver range-gate location in the M-mode.

(most often the heart), showing echo-source motion over time. As noted before, motion characteristics and heart anatomy permit an operator to decide where the beam is pointing. Still, exact positioning is difficult because this display form carries a lot of information about motion, but little information about anatomy. Nevertheless, an M-mode trace is still a useful tool in positioning a Doppler sample volume. Importantly, the M-mode image remains truly simultaneous with the Doppler display, which is the organizational hallmark of a true duplex system.

Doppler signal processing in an M/Q system looks like that in any coherent, pulsed-Doppler system (see Chapter 6). For example, the receiver often has an adjustable range gate to limit and define the source of the Doppler echo signals. This gate appears on the M/Q display as a straight line (Fig. 8-3).

After Doppler signal separation at the QPD, the system detects and analyses the Doppler shift frequencies in each direction channel. In its original form, signal analysis came from listening to the Doppler sounds. Soon this was followed by additional analysis based on the zero-crossing detector.[3] Fast Fourier transform analysis[4] powers the current designs.

The M/Q system began as a stand-alone device but soon became part of the next generation of real-time duplex systems. It remains part of many duplex systems designed for echocardiography.

Time-Share Duplex Imaging

A duplex system that must image in real-time and also carry out Doppler interrogations is simply unable to do both at the same time. These conflicting operations must share time. Because conventional imaging and Doppler processing have conflicting transmitting needs, imaging and Doppler functions use different transmitters. The real-time image, for example, uses a sharp electrical spike to excite the transducer. Doppler excitation, on the other hand, comes from a coherent gated transmitter. In simple terms, a time-shared system does some imaging, then some Doppler, then imaging and so on.

On the receiving side, the transducer sees the incoherent ultrasound burst from the imaging transmitter and the coherent bursts from the Doppler transmitter. These two sorts of signals do not mix well within the tissues or the signal processing. In addition, the transmitting power levels for the two are often very different. Doppler echo signals, for example, come from backscattering groups of RBCs, and these signals are typically 40 to 60 dB below the tissue signals.[5] To obtain adequate penetration and maintain a good Doppler signal-to-noise ratio, the Doppler output powers can be quite large. Indeed, they can be 10 to 20 times larger than output powers typical of imaging systems alone.

The internal organization of these systems is now rather well integrated, but early systems comprised several separate subsystems. They shared only the same transducer and a master timer to control the time-sharing events. Some current duplex systems still show this high-level separation beneath the smooth skin of new industrial packaging.

Imaging and CW Doppler Processing

Combining CW Doppler functions and real-time imaging produces the very simple duplex system shown in Figure 8-4. The transducer is often a linear array with a separate, outboard CW Doppler transducer attached to the real-time scanhead. Within the image is a Doppler direction line that shows where the beam points within the image-scanning plane. Although the CW Doppler transducer is movable in some designs, it is more often fixed.

Moving a separate Doppler beam inside an image requires a position encoder on the Doppler transducer. The encoder tracks the position of the Doppler beam and links this motion to a cursor on the display (Fig. 8-5). Typically, activating the Doppler operating mode freezes the real-time image. This means that the operator must hold the

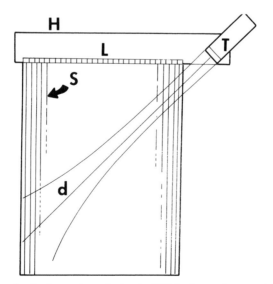

Figure 8-4   CW Doppler duplex system. A simple CW duplex system consists of a CW Doppler transducer (*T*) mechanically coupled with a linear array (*L*). *H* is the housing that joins the two together. The Doppler beam (*d*) is fixed and crosses the linear array scan lines (*S*).

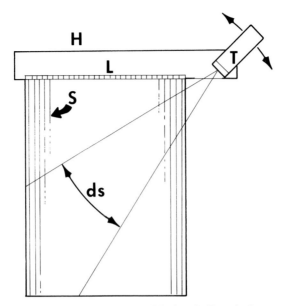

Figure 8-5   Movable CW Doppler duplex system. Moving the Doppler beam over a sector (*ds*) re-quires an encoder to translate beam position into signals for positioning the image cursor. *H* is a common housing, *L* is the linear array, and *S* is the linear array scan lines.

scanhead very still while manipulating the Doppler beam into position. In contrast, a fixed Doppler transducer requires that the operator manipulate the whole scanhead to image the vessel and at the same time, maneuver the vessel into the CW Doppler beam.

This combination of imaging and CW Doppler functions has several traditional weaknesses. The first is the alignment of the CW Doppler transducer within the scanning plane of the real-time linear array. The Doppler beam must be in the real-time scan plane throughout the imaging field of view. Maintaining this alignment for an outboard system requires a large, strong transducer attachment. The attachment design becomes more difficult if the Doppler transducer must also move. In addition, a CW Doppler device cannot separate echo sources along its beam, which markedly reduces some of the benefits of joining it to a real-time image. It is a strange situation to see more than one vessel within an image and still be unable to localize the Doppler signals to a single one.

The Doppler output for this form of duplex is typically an analog "mean" frequency waveform and Doppler sounds. Some of the more complete Doppler designs may include a conventional spectral display, with a zero-crossing detector or a fast Fourier transform device. These systems can handle only those few tasks that fit into the limited image allowed by Doppler beam geometry and display. From a clinical point of view, the ability of the system to separate one vessel from another is compromised. Imaging the internal and external carotid artery at the same time, for example, would make it difficult to separate the two vessels. Figure 8-6 shows the nature of this problem. It was these sorts of limitations and problems that caused this particular duplex system to vanish from the clinical scene.

Imaging and Pulsed Doppler Processing

The first imaging and pulsed-Doppler duplex systems included a mechanical sector scanner and a pulsed-Doppler transducer.[1] Initially, the transducer was outboard with a

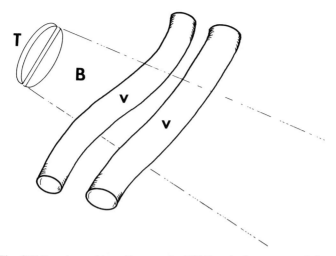

Figure 8-6   The CW Doppler problem. Because the CW Doppler has no range information, all vessels (*v*) that are in the beam (*B*) at the same time produce signals. Or conversely, if one vessel is occluded and flow exists in the other, the occlusion remains hidden. *T* is the transducer.

small lever to position the ultrasound beam and sample volume.[6] This arrangement appears in Figure 8-7. In contrast, most of the current systems have a more integrated approach, using either the same transducer for both Doppler and imaging, or a separate outboard Doppler transducer.

   A common transducer, separate power requirements, and different needs for transmitting coherency combine to force this duplex design into time sharing. Interrogation begins by using the real-time image to locate the vessel or heart chamber of interest. After locating the vessel, the operator uses the pulsed-Doppler function to examine flow within the vessel or heart chamber. Doppler interrogation in a time-sharing format, however, requires a frozen real-time image. With a frozen image to

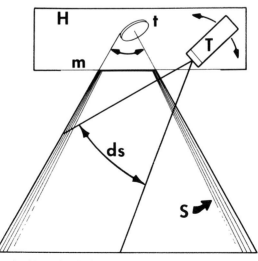

Figure 8-7   Outboard pulsed Doppler duplex system. The first pulsed Doppler duplex system used a mechanical sector scan (*t*) for the image and an outboard Doppler transducer (*T*) that moved over a sector (*ds*). *S* is the sector scanlines, *H* is the common housing, and *m* is a sonolucent membrane, maintaining a fluid interior to the housing.

guide the way, the operator positions the sample volume indicator along a movable on-screen cursor line (Fig. 8-8). The receiver range gate location graphically appears on the cursor line as a slash, dot, or sometimes, a pair of lines.

Although the vessel is steady in the image, patient movement and respiration, movement of the sonographer's hand, or simple misalignment between Doppler beam and vessel can all cause problems. Because the image is frozen on the last real-time image, the movement is not detectable. Often, movement will cause the Doppler spectrum to change, but most users rely heavily on a steady patient and scanning hand.

As we noted earlier, the different transmitter timing and energy needs for a coherent Doppler transmission force a separation of transmitters, one for imaging and another for Doppler. In some cases, the Doppler transmitter can operate at a frequency lower than the imaging frequency, using the same broad-bandwidth transducer. Most systems, however, use the same frequency for both.

Moving to a lower Doppler carrier frequency improves the penetration of the ultrasound into the tissue. Unfortunately, it also decreases the backscatter of ultrasound from the RBCs. To compensate, many of these systems use a much higher output power to get flow information from the more distant blood vessels. The lower carrier frequency also proportionately lowers the Doppler shift frequencies for all blood flow velocities. Thus, the higher Doppler frequencies associated with stenosis are decreased, and many of the lower velocities do not appear. The disappearing low velocities can create another problem.

Many flow problems involve slow-moving blood and that means low Doppler shift frequencies. Indeed, the frequencies may be below the lowest frequency threshold for the sonograph. Simple calculations using the Doppler equation show the following relationship: if the lowest velocity a 7.5-MHz Doppler can depict is 6 cm/s, then moving the carrier to 5.0 MHz increases that minimum to 9 cm/s. Under the same conditions, a 3.0-MHz carrier increases the minimum to 15 cm/s.

Linear phased arrays are also excellent candidates for a duplex system. It turns out that many of the Doppler transmitting needs are already part of the phased array.

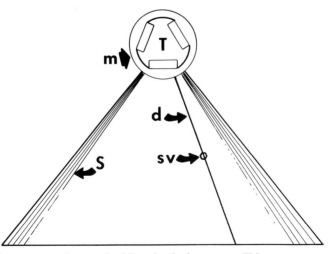

Figure 8-8   Common transducer, pulsed Doppler duplex system. This system uses a motor driven (*m*) rotating scan head (*T*). Actuating the Doppler function requires freezing the scanhead along a particular scanline (*d*) and moving the sample volume (*sv*) to the right position. The Doppler cursor (*d*) always aligns with one of the imaging scan lines (*S*). The lack of any image update during Doppler activation requires scanning with a steady hand.

Color Section

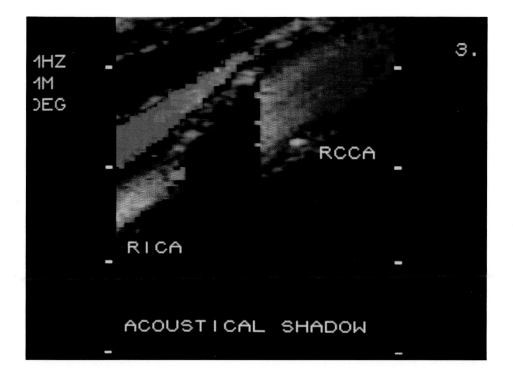

Figure 3-13 Example of soft-tissue acoustical shadow. In this angiodynogram, calcified plaque on the anterior wall of the vessel casts a shadow (absence of color) across the vessel and the soft tissue behind the vessel. RCCA, right common carotid artery; RICA, internal carotid artery.

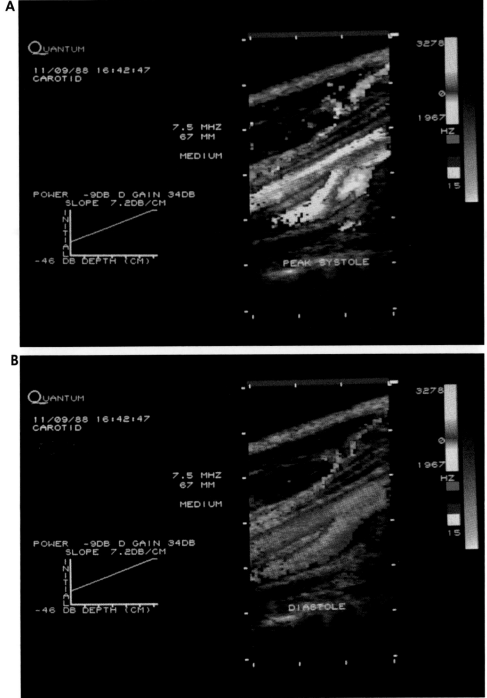

Figure 4-17 Angiodynograms of flow separation in a normal carotid bulb. **A,** During systole, the reversed flow in the carotid bulb appears *blue* in the *red* flow pattern. The *whiter* segments of the red flow pattern indicate the major streamlines. **B,** In diastole, the pressure gradient between the separation zone and common carotid decreases. The separation flow is then very small or zero, and appears *black* in the image.

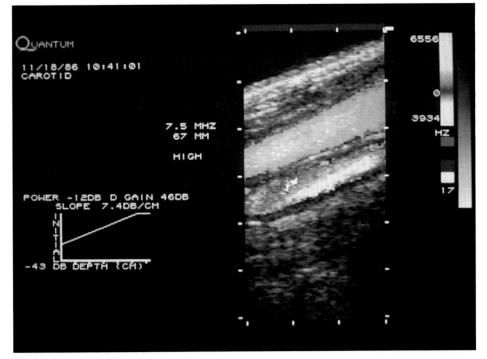

Figure 5-7 Non-axial streamlines in a vessel. The *lighter* portions of the *red* arterial flow pattern show a major streamline traversing the vessel lumen. In this example, the major streamline deviates more than 15° from parallel to the vessel wall. Measurements of Doppler shift frequencies at 60° would have an error of nearly 48% from the true value, whether measured upstream or downstream.

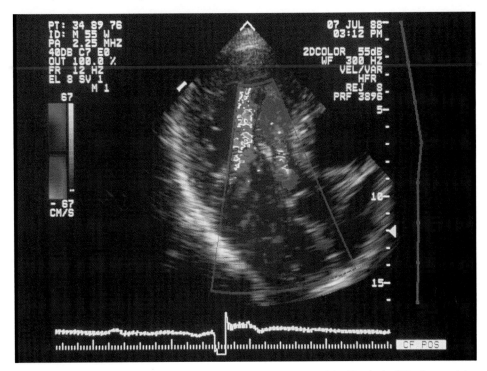

Figure 8-14 A color flow image of the heart. Apical view of the left ventricle. Ventricular filling is toward the transducer (*red*) with a small amount of turbulence (*green*). The filling curls in the apex of the venticle and flows toward the left ventricular outflow tract away from the transducer (*blue*). (Courtesy of ATL, Inc., Bothell, Washington.)

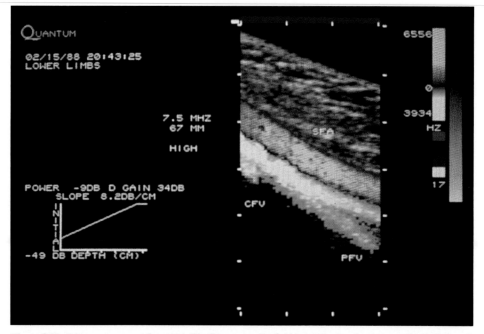

Figure 8-17   Linear array scan of a vessel. The linear scanning field is appropriate for correct color depiction of flow events in a vessel. In this setting, changes in color within the flow field can represent changes in the flow direction within the vessel. This superficial femoral artery (*red*) shows the same color for flow within the vessel, representing a normal arterial flow pattern. The *blue* vessel is the femoral vein.

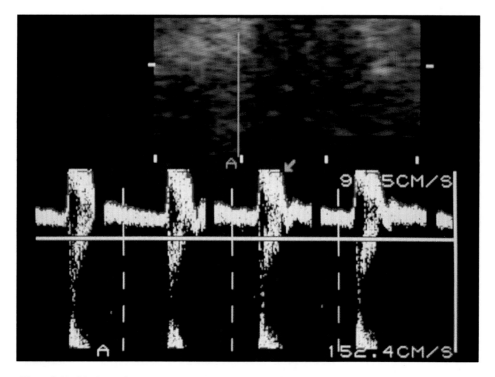

Figure 8-21   Maximum frequency line aliasing. Aliasing interferes with measuring events in the spectrum. In this example, the maximum frequency (*green line*) does not show the complete wave form. It truncates at the limit (*small green arrow*). Measurements of wave form pulsatility would be in error on this spectrum. *A* is the spectrum cursor.

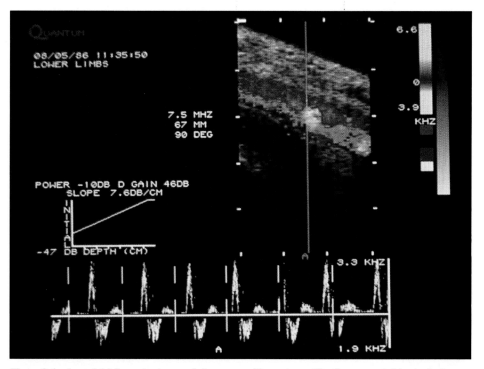

Figure 9-4 Superficial femoral artery angiodynogram with spectrum. The flow reversal (*blue* in the image, downward stroke in the spectrum) in a normal femoral artery is the result of reflections from distal changes in hydraulic impedance. When the reflections first arrive, they do not involve the whole vessel (the *blue* flow reversal in the *red* forward flow). A is the spectral sampling cursor.

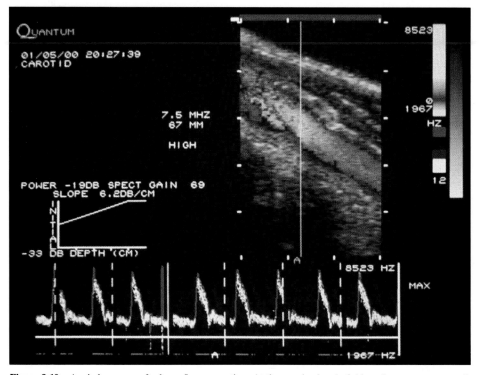

Figure 9-10 Angiodynogram of a large flow separation. At the proximal end of this endarterectomy, a small posterior lip is deviating flow toward the anterior wall. The flow deviation produces a larger flow separation and reversal in systole (*blue*). A is the spectrum cursor. The time course of the flow is shown in the spectrum below.

Figure 9-5A, B overleaf

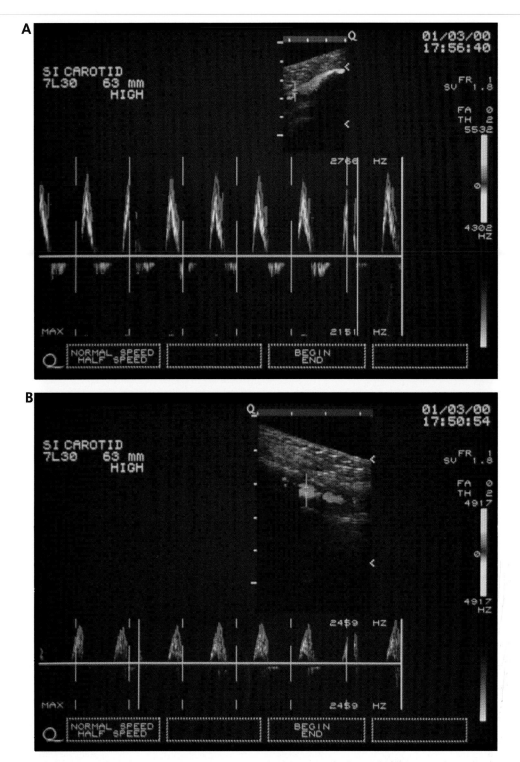

Figure 9-5 Differences in wave forms proximal and distal to a stenosis. Lower limb flow wave forms appear different when proximal and distal to a stenosis. **A,** Proximal flow shows a biphasic wave form with steep acceleration and deceleration phases. The steepness comes from high distal resistance. **B,** Distal flow shows a monophasic, rounded wave form with lower acceleration, deceleration, and peak flow values. The *green* in both examples marks the maximum frequency.

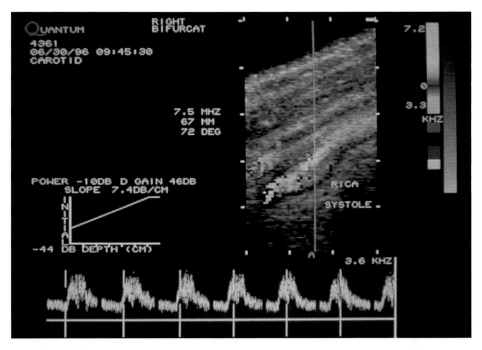

Figure 9-11 Angiodynogram of a normal carotid bulb with disturbed flow. The flow disorganization in this carotid bulb appears as frequency broadening in the spectrum. *A* is the spectrum cursor.

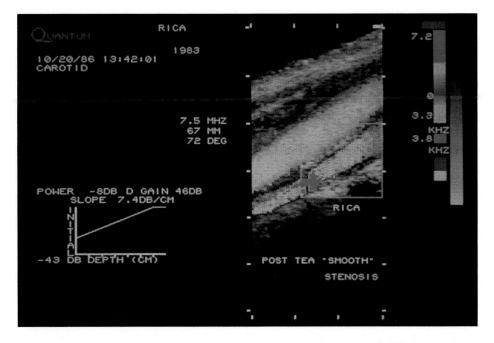

Figure 9-12 Angiodynogram of smooth wall stenosis. This example shows restenosis following an endarterectomy. Walls are smooth and the lumen is narrow, generating uniform acceleration without flow disturbances. The *green* region in the vessel marks the higher Doppler frequencies and velocities in the color flow image.

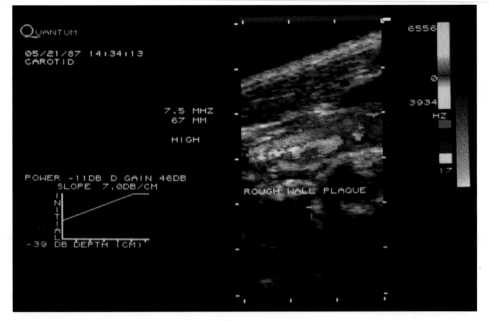

Figure 9-13 Angiodynogram of rough wall flow. Wall irregularities, both large and small, cause the flow stream-lines to tumble. This alters color and saturation at each of these changes in flow direction. The *blue elements* in the *red arterial field* show each of these reversal sites.

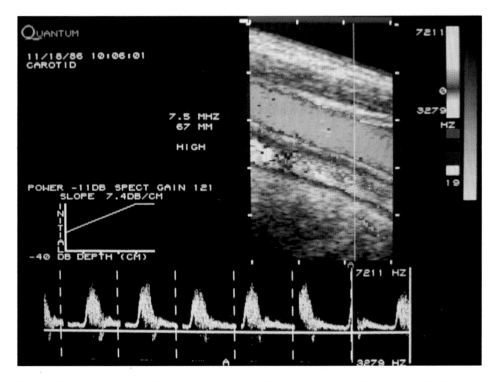

Figure 9-22 Angiodynogram of common carotid artery with in-line turbulence. The hallmark of in-line tur-bulence is the breakup of streamlines without compromising bulk flow. In this unobstructed carotid artery, in-line turbulence creates a *mottled appearance* to the flow pattern, and spectral broadening in the spectral recording.

The linear phased array is made of many individually unfocused transducers, arranged into a linear geometry. Because the array must work as if it were a single source of ultrasound, the timing among the array elements is both fine and critical. Many of the phased arrays use a sine wave to excite each of the transducer elements into vibration because this method provides better timing and control than a conventional spike transmitter. Each excitation voltage, however, must arrive at a specific time to combine the emission from each of the transducer elements into a single ultrasound beam. Both timing and delay come from delay lines that control the transmitter voltages that reach the transducers. The focused beam forms a coherent burst of ultrasonic waves during transmission. Such a coherent burst is key to a coherent pulsed-Doppler system.

Timing and delay in the phased array not only allow beam focusing, they permit beam steering. The beam steering generates a sector-scanning field. Beam steering also requires additional changes in timing, but as a beam moves off center, new radiation patterns appear. These so-called grating lobes appear along with the major lobe as shown in Figure 8-9. Grating lobes from a phased array degrade both imaging and Doppler functions by making the sample volume appear very large close to the transducer (Fig. 8-10).

Nevertheless, one real benefit in duplex imaging with a phased array is the steady lines of sight formed by electronic beam steering. It is easy to select one line of sight for the Doppler beam position and update the remainder of the image. Each single phased-array beam forms a steady line-of-sight position. Updating the image does not require physical transducer movement as in a mechanical sector scanner. In addition, electronic focusing can work on both transmitting (zonal) and receiving (dynamic) sides of the pulse-listen cycle. The result can be a very small sample volume over a large part of the scanning field.

In general, the strengths of duplex pulsed-Doppler systems reside in three areas. First, a pulsed-Doppler system can produce a better form of time sharing than a CW

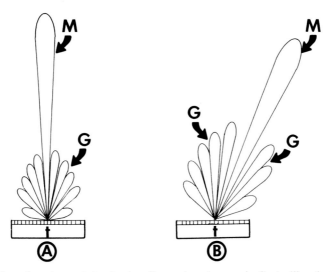

Figure 8-9   Beam focusing and steering in a linear phased array. **A,** Controlling the timing among the transducer elements (*t*) produces a main beam (*M*) with grating lobes (*G*). **B,** Beam steering, shifts the main beam position but the grating lobes increase in amplitude and number. The best focusing occurs when the beam is perpendicular to the array and the grating lobes can be reduced.

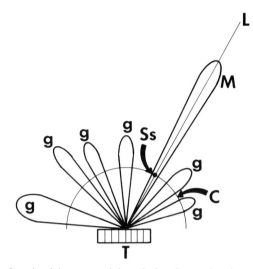

Figure 8-10   Effects of grating lobes on spatial resolution. Increasing the grating lobes (*g*) can confuse event sampling. In this example, flow events in the sample site (*Ss*) can be hidden by flow in any grating lobe, at the range shown as a common time arc (*C*). *M* is the main lobe, *L* is the display line of sight, and *T* is the transducer array.

Doppler system. Second, the imaging updating can be quite fast, which makes sample volume placement more accurate. Third, a pulsed-Doppler format with range gating uniquely defines the location of the Doppler signal source.

The weakness of the mechanical duplex systems are many: a difficulty in aligning the Doppler ultrasound beam in the scanning field; a changing angle between the image and the Doppler line of sight as the Doppler beam swings through an arc; an inherent inflexibility common to outboard systems; and using the system requires additional experience and skill when the Doppler mode freezes the B-mode image.

Many of these difficulties, however, either vanish or are minimized with advanced, true duplex systems.

Advanced True Duplex Systems

Two forms of advance duplex imaging exist for the cardiovascular system: color flow imaging for the heart and vascular system, and angiodynography for the vascular system.[7] They have similar images that provide a color depiction of flow with a gray-scale depiction of surrounding soft tissue. Despite their look-alike images, these systems use different signal-processing techniques, which are reflected in their names.

Collecting the Data

The advanced techniques that create a flow image depend upon a unique method of gathering information from the scanning field. Parallel signal processing within the sonograph collects amplitude, phase, and frequency information from the echo signals. This data gathering can happen at different times (asynchronous processing) or at the same time (synchronous processing). In an ideal system, Doppler sampling points in a scanning field would map onto the display as image pixels (Fig. 8-11).

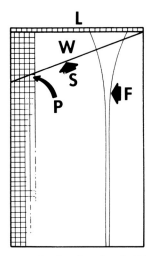

Figure 8-11   Sampling for synchronous color flow imaging. In this system, the linear array (*L*) forms dynamically focused beams (*F*) that scan down the array. The image is separated into sampling sites (*P*) approximately one wavelength long. *W* is a stand-off wedge to provide a Doppler angle, and *S* is the skin-wedge interface. This synchronous sampling organization is used in angiodynography.

In asynchronous processing, the system first gathers some gray-scale information, then some Doppler information. The practical aspects of first gathering and then processing a large amount of signal information from deep vessels can make equal image and Doppler spatial resolution impossible. For example, an image might contain high-resolution gray scale and a much coarser two-dimensional portrayal of blood movement. The sampling for blood flow is less exact because it requires much larger sampling sites and intervals.

The block diagram of a synchronous, generic, real-time, color flow-mapping system (Fig. 8-12) shows the control of the transmitted burst for phase and frequency content. The same things happen in any coherent Doppler system. Unlike a simple Doppler system, the returning echo signal splits into two separate processing channels. One channel detects the echo signal for amplitude; the other passes first through a QPD that detects motion and separates this motion into forward and reverse channels (Fig. 8-12). After normal Doppler detection and spectral analysis, the system codes the Doppler signals into color and then merges the gray-scale (amplitude) portion of the signal path at the scan converter.

The merger of two sorts of signals is based on specific decision rules about placing color in the digital scan converter. For example, choosing to color a particular pixel or not depends on how much motion is present within the corresponding Doppler sampling region. It also depends on the amplitude of the Doppler echo signal returning from that same sample site. Ultimately, the decision-making rules should reject noise and motion ambiguity and still accurately separate moving blood from stationary tissue.

The front panel controls on the machine, which set up the color portrayal of flow, can change these rules. Large vessels with fast-moving blood that sits close to the skin will have different rules from very small vessels with slow-moving blood that sit deep in the tissue. To obtain the most accurate color images of flow, the user must set up the color display for the type of vessels being scanned.

Asynchronous signal processing produces a very similar image to synchronous

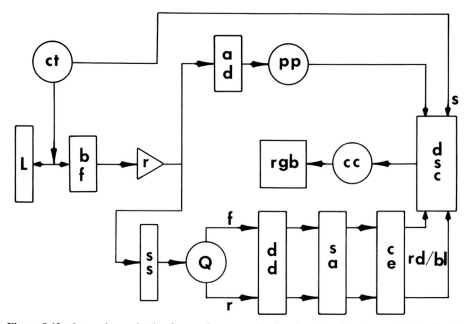

Figure 8-12   Internal organization for synchronous color flow imaging. See the text for details. *L* is the linear array, *ct* is the coherent transmitter, *bf* is the beam forming elements, and *r* is a common receiver. The signal branches into two pathways. The image pathway: *ad* is the amplitude detector, and *pp* is gray scale post processing. The Doppler pathway: *ss* separates moving from stationary echo signals, *Q* is the quadrature phase detector, *dd* is Doppler detection in forward (*f*) and reverse (*r*) channels, *sa* is an on-line spectral analysis, and *ce* is color encoding (red and blue, rd/bl). Both channels enter the digital scan converter (*dsc*), continue to color coding (*cc*) and finally go to an red/green/blue (*rgb*) graphics monitor. *s* is a synchronization signal for the *dsc*.

processing, but the internal organization is quite different. Figure 8-13 shows the typical organization of an asynchronous color system. Because of the different signal-processing needs, the imaging and Doppler signal paths have only the transducer as a common element. The functions within each portion of this system are the same as in the synchronous system. Gray-scale information will still come from amplitude detection; Doppler information will still come from coherent pulsed-Doppler processing.

Dealing with Color Parameters

Introducing color codes to depict Doppler shift frequencies means having to deal with the physical parameters of color. In general, a color has three components: hue, brightness, and saturation.

Hue expresses the color itself, that is, the wavelength or frequency of the electromagnetic energy. The wave frequency produces the biological effect we perceive as color. For example, blue is a shorter wavelength and higher frequency than red. Changing hue means changing the wavelength or frequency of the light. Thus, a change from red to blue is a change in hue.

Brightness deals with the changing intensity of a color, i.e., how much energy the color contains. The brightness of a color can change without changing either the wavelength or the saturation. A good example of changing brightness is seen when the illumination onto a color swatch is altered: as the illumination decreases, the color appears darker, but the frequency (wavelength) and saturation are unchanged.

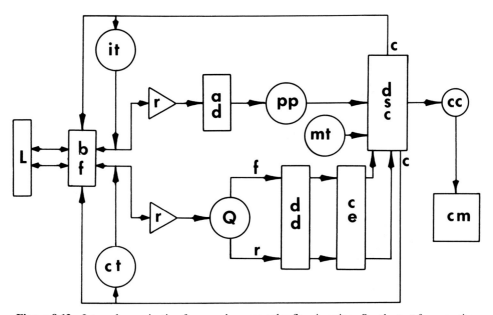

Figure 8-13 Internal organization for asynchronous color flow imaging. See the text for operating details. *L* is the linear array; *bf* are beam-forming elements. On the image side, the image transmitter is *it*, *r* is the receiver, *ad* is the amplitude detector, and *pp* is preprocessing, including analog-to-digital conversion. *dsc* is the digital scan converter. On the Doppler side, *r* is the receiver, *Q* is the quadrature phase detector, *f* and *r* are forward and reverse channels, *dd* is Doppler detection, and *ce* is color encoding. *ct* is the coherent transmitter. *mt* is the main timing and control, with control signals, *c*, to transmitters and beamformers for each image. *cc* is the color encoder, and *cm* is a color monitor.

Color saturation describes color purity. If a color is 100% saturated, then it contains no other colors; it is 100% pure. Decreasing the saturation adds more whiteness into the color. Visually, the color shades to a whiter appearance. For example, a color saturation starting at 100% saturation would show a deep red; with decreasing saturation, the color along the bar changes to lighter and lighter reds.

The Benefits of Color

The use of color coding information in medical imaging has had a mixed history. The images generated by color-coding B-mode, nuclear medicine, and computed tomography are not particularly new. Even spectral recordings have been color coded. In general, these uses of color have not conveyed new or different information from that already carried in the gray-scale image. As a result, color often appears to be a gimmick rather than an additional means of conveying information.

Two primary tasks in any diagnostic imaging system are to detect disease and provide some means of evaluating its extent. Color flow imaging offers a means of rapidly detecting the flow abnormalities that indicate disease, such as the disruption of streamlines, the formation of eddy currents and vortices, and the acceleration of stenosis. Color also provides rapid detection and localization of flow within an image, and finally, the direction of that flow with respect to the transducer.

In the end, color will add enough new information to an image to make the detection of flow abnormalities fast and easy, but events within the image may not be simple. The presence and distribution of color enables a direct evaluation of stenotic disease in vessels and valvular incompetence in the heart. Reading the image, however, still requires an understanding of how the system makes the color image and the hemodynamics associated with normal and abnormal physiology. Nevertheless, the two-dimensional depiction of flow patterns permits a more accurate estimate of flow velocities within a vessel lumen and through heart valves.

Color Flow Imaging

At the center of color flow imaging is parallel signal processing of echo signals for amplitude, phase, and frequency. The amplitude information becomes a real-time, gray-scale image. At the same time, the system must identify moving tissue, ignore this movement, and portray the tissue in gray scale.

The phase information is a primary indication of motion, and based on phase changes, the system separates an echo signal into forward and reverse channels. Signals in these channels become colors, most often red and blue, that depict both the presence and direction of the motion.

Coding Doppler frequency information involves additional signal processing. For example, increasing a Doppler shift frequency could shift the color hue (for example, red would move toward orange with increasing frequency, and blue toward green). In contrast, the coding could also be as simple as changing the saturation of a color to represent frequency. One color flow system uses three colors, red, green, and blue, to express the direction, velocity, and variance of blood flow[8] (Fig. 8-14, see color section between pp. 116 and 117). In this system, red is forward flow, blue is reverse flow. Turbulence appears in green, giving a forward turbulence a yellow color and reverse turbulence a blue-green color. A changing frequency or velocity then appears as a changing brightness.

The task of this system design is to depict vessel or heart anatomy and the physiology of blood flow at the same time. Central to this task is an adequate separation of tissue from blood movement. This is more difficult when the tissue movements are both fast and complex, as in the heart.

The basic operating character of the linear phased array makes color flow imaging an excellent addition to this sort of echocardiograph. At the outset, the phased array steers its beam in fixed steps through a sector. Each electronic beam formation and position is fixed and exactly the same on each image frame. In contrast, a mechanical sector scanner has a continuously moving beam that is unsuitable for easy Doppler signal processing. The fixed-beam position assures a static line of sight to gather Doppler information. Phased array transmission is also coherent for both imaging and Doppler processing. This permits using changing phase and frequency to gather information about echo-source motion. Furthermore, because this coherency exists throughout the image, simultaneous (true duplex) Doppler signal processing is possible.

The phased array, however, creates a sector-scanning field. Such a scanning process constantly changes the Doppler angle along a linear flow pattern. The changing Doppler angle imposes a set of color changes that can make detection of abnormal flow patterns more difficult. In this situation, a linear flow pattern will change color, or even lose color, depending upon its location in the sector-scanning field (Fig. 8-15). Changing colors then represent either an alteration in scan angle or flow pattern or both. The difficulty is separating these two effects from one another. This geometric interaction between flow direction and beam orientation requires careful consideration to identify the actual flow pattern. Vessels really require a different scanning pattern.

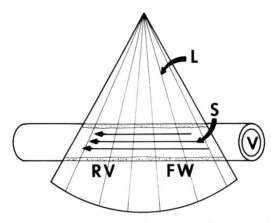

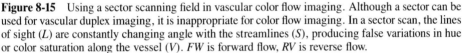

Figure 8-15   Using a sector scanning field in vascular color flow imaging. Although a sector can be used for vascular duplex imaging, it is inappropriate for color flow imaging. In a sector scan, the lines of sight (*L*) are constantly changing angle with the streamlines (*S*), producing false variations in hue or color saturation along the vessel (*V*). *FW* is forward flow, *RV* is reverse flow.

In echocardiography, the phased array sector works quite well. First, the scanning positions for color are not the same for traditional heart imaging. For example, a parasternal image places the ultrasound beams perpendicular to the flow pattern, removing useful Doppler information (cos θ becomes zero). As a result, color flow imaging is typically from an apical or subcostal position that places the blood motion more parallel to the ultrasound beams (Fig. 8-16). Because the cos θ is a slow-changing function near 0°, this imaging position diminishes the effects of sector field on the color pattern.

Angiodynography

Angiodynography is a new word in ultrasound. *Angio* comes from a root word meaning vessel, and *dynography* means the depiction or measurement of dynamics. Angiodynography, then, is a portrayal of flow dynamics within a vessel. In its current form, angiodynography examines the vascular compartments with greater detail than earlier color flow imaging designs. The available transducer frequencies include 7.5 MHz, 5.0 MHz, and 3.0 MHz. Peripheral vascular imaging uses much higher Doppler carrier frequencies than typical of cardiac color flow imaging.[8] These higher frequencies give better spatial (axial and lateral) resolution for both the imaging and Doppler signal processing. Current signal processing provides the same sampling rate along each line of sight for both gray-scale imaging and Doppler.[7]

In general, vessels in the neck, arms, and legs are closer to the transducer than the deeper parts of the heart. This means shorter fields of view and much higher frame rates for angiodynography than in typical color flow imaging. These higher frame rates give a better depiction of flow patterns in vessels throughout the cardiac cycle. The faster frame rates, however, require faster calculations of spectral frequency components during the composition of each image frame. This high-speed processing is a central need in angiodynography.

Most vessels of interest in the body are parallel or nearly parallel to the skin surface. And although these vessels are not entirely straight, small segments are linear or nearly so. This an ideal situation for a linear array that can supply a Doppler scanning angle either through beam steering or a wedge. With a constant scanning angle from the

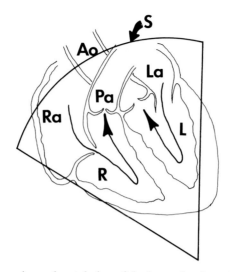

Figure 8-16   Flow patterns in a subcostal view of the heart. A subcostal sector view of the heart places a lot of the flow pattern parallel to the ultrasound beams. This makes the sector geometry a good choice for cardiac color flow imaging. *S* is the sector, *L* and *R* are left and right ventricles, *Pa* is pulmonary artery, *La* is left atrium, *Ao* is aorta, and *Ra* is right atrium.

linear array intercepting linear vessel segments, color changes can directly represent flow disturbances (Fig. 8-17, see color section between pp. 116 and 117).

In this situation, movement in the same direction within a vessel will produce the same color. At the same time, flow deviations within the vessel that change direction relative to the transducer cause a color change. In other words, color changes represent flow changes. These changes can be due to disease or the normal variations in anatomy and hemodynamics produced by a complex vascular system.

Determining how much disease exists within vessels, such as the extracranial arteries, centers on three conditions. They are also risk conditions for the vascular system: percent stenosis, vessel wall condition, and vessel intimal condition.

Separating arterial disease into these particular segments is more a didactic tool than the way we might think about the problem. It is a way of understanding the role of the technology in asking the questions. For example, stenosis causes both an acceleration in blood velocity and a color-defined, flow channel narrowing. The system gray scale will portray the mass that is leading to a lumen narrowing. And finally, the color and gray-scale separation at the blood-tissue interface will show the pattern of flow over the interface.

On a practical basis, the investigation with angiodynography would start with a search for plaque or a thrombus by looking for their effects on flow. And if a mass is impeding flow, the final expression of this impediment might be a statement of percent stenosis. Now, our original three risk questions become more practical: Is blood flow being obstructed? If so, what is causing the obstruction? And finally, is the flow over the obstruction smooth or complicated?

In the end, stenosis, wall condition, and intimal condition are not independent of one another. And no single condition is enough to accurately predict the progression of vascular disease and ensuing complications such as stroke or claudication. Of the three, the most difficult evaluation is the intimal condition because it requires the depiction of very low amplitude flow signals in the presence of very large tissue signals.

The conditions for signal separation at the boundary between blood and vessel wall are not the best for signal processing. The vessel wall signals may be 40 to 60 dB larger than the signals from the adjacent RBCs. All these signals sum together creating large, phase-changing signals that do not represent blood flow. The system task is to separate the blood signals from the wall signals.

The first step in improving the separation is to use smaller sample volumes. Second, the sampling over the vessel and at the vessel wall must be small enough to depict small flow changes. Third, the internal signal separation must be good enough to keep the spatial separation accurate to plus-or-minus one sampling site. Satisfying these three demands can give a system the ability to depict very small flow disturbances at the intimal boundary. These disturbances will often represent intimal surface roughness.

High Frequency Aliasing

Within a process in which a continuous signal is discretely sampled to follow its changes lies a hidden source of error and uncertainty. This uncertainty is high-frequency aliasing, and for the unsuspecting, it can be a source of confusion and ambiguous results.

Very likely, our first introduction to motion aliasing was not in an engineering or physics class but at the movies. As the stagecoach raced by, the coach wheels appeared to be rotating backward rather than forward. This illogical situation is the result of a mismatch between the sampling rate (the number of still frames per second used in making the film) and the motion of the wheels and spokes. The first clue to the rules governing aliasing occurs when the coach slows. As the wheels slow down, they gradually stop moving backward and start turning forward again.

In Doppler ultrasound, a similar event occurs when a pulsed-Doppler system samples the motion of an echo source. For the pulsed Doppler system, the motion is being sampled at the system's pulse repetition frequency (PRF), as shown in Figure 8-18. When the Doppler shift frequency exceeds PRF divided by two, high-frequency aliasing changes the apparent phase and frequency of the Doppler shift frequency. On a spectral display, the aliased frequencies disappear from the top of one directional chan-

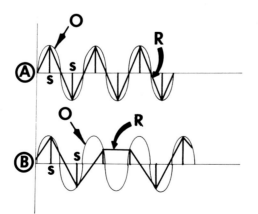

Figure 8-18   Signal sampling and high-frequency aliasing. One way to understand the sampling problem is to look at a sine wave (*O*) that is being sampled (*s*). **A,** The sampling rate is twice the object frequency (*O*), producing a new signal (*R*) that contains the basic frequency information. **B,** Not sampling often enough produces a distorted result (*R*) that can look like a lower frequency (take on an "alias").

nel and reappear as lower frequencies in the opposite channel. For example, if aliasing occurs in the forward spectrum, the aliased signals appear in the reverse spectrum. Figure 8-19 shows an example of high-frequency aliasing.

A rigorous look at the sampling problem shows that the ability to follow a signal disappears when the signal frequency exceeds the sampling frequency limit. This sampling limit is the Nyquist limit,[4] and under most conditions, it is half the sampling frequency. For a typical ultrasound system sampling motion at the PRF, the Nyquist limit becomes the PRF divided by two. This limit is a rigorous rule under most signal processing circumstances in ultrasound.

Aliasing is a problem in Doppler ultrasound because it masks information. If aliasing occurs in a noisy Doppler spectrum, for example, the peak frequencies can alias into the noise and clutter of spectral broadening. Automatic calculations of peak frequency parameters have no value in these situations as well.

Aliasing can also make it quite difficult to identify the form of the flow pattern over time. This is especially true in systems that offer only an analog signal output rather than a complete spectrum. In color flow imaging and angiodynography, aliasing can create color patterns that hide the true flow pattern.

Aliasing can also be apparent and not real. This occurs when a peak frequency on a spectrum exceeds the display limits but not necessarily the Nyquist limit. The first move for a sonographer suspecting that aliasing is occurring is to change the spectral display range to make sure that the aliasing is real and not simply a display limitation. An alternative is to shift the spectral signal baseline, also known as a zero-shift or

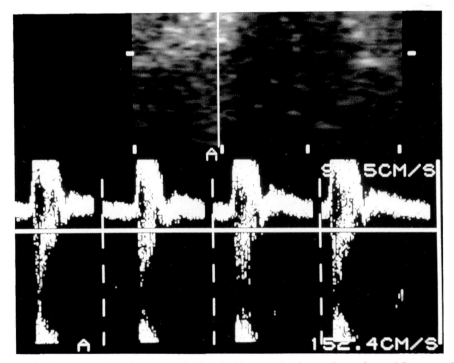

Figure 8-19   Spectral high-frequency aliasing. In this example, the maximum forward flow exceeds the upper frequency limit and appears in the opposite channel as a lower frequency. *A* is the spectral cursor.

baseline control. None of these controls, however, is changing the relationship between the Doppler shift frequencies and the Nyquist limit. Only the spectral display range is changing.

Aliasing is more evident on a complete spectral display than on a single element display showing just the mean or maximum frequency.[9] This is especially true when the mean value calculation is double sided, that is, the mean frequency considers both forward (above the zero line) and reverse (below the zero line) Doppler shift frequencies. Single line aliasing is shown in Figure 8-20.

Some Solutions for Aliasing

Aliasing becomes a problem when it interferes with the diagnostic function of a sonograph. For example, aliasing can alter calculations that estimate the amount of disease that may be present (Fig. 8-21, see color section between pp. 116 and 117). The direct way of dealing with aliasing is to increase the effective Nyquist limit.

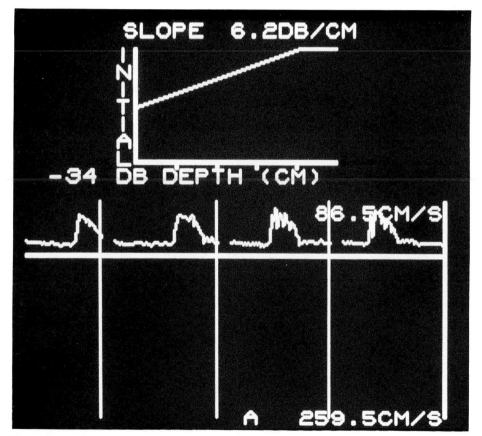

Figure 8-20 Spectral single-line aliasing. Aliasing appears differently when the spectrum is a single frequency (line). In this example, the two flow cycles on the *left* are not aliasing, but the two on the *right* are. The "noise" on the waveform comes from the aliasing, which is otherwise invisible. As a result, detecting aliasing in a spectrum requires seeing the complete spectrum and not a single frequency.

Using Complex Mathematics

A look at the theoretical frequency response from digital sampling shows why the sampling bandwidth is limited to the sampling frequency divided by two. If the sampling occurs on a real number, then a sampled power spectrum is symmetrical about the zero value.[9] In this configuration, the effective bandwidth is half the sampling frequency. Chapter 7 reviews this event in detail (see Fig. 7-17, A and B).

If, on the other hand, sampling occurs on a mathematically complex number (consisting of real and imaginary parts), then the power spectrum is not symmetrical about the zero value.[9] Moving the sampling bandwidth as if it were a filter creates an operating bandwidth equal to the sampling frequency.[10] The results of spectral analysis on a complex function are shown in Figure 7-17 (C and D).

One way, then, to remove the Nyquist limit in Doppler signal processing is to use complex signal analysis. The result is an aliasing limit at PRF.

Increasing the PRF

Another method of increasing the Nyquist limit is simply to increase the system's PRF. This approach forms the so-called high-PRF systems. The PRF increase goes in discrete steps, however. Each increase must be an exact multiple of the lowest PRF in the system, which is determined by the system's display depth. For example, if a sonograph uses a 4-KHz PRF, the first increase would be 8 KHz (twice the base PRF), then 12 KHz (three times the base PRF), then 16 KHz (four times the base PRF), etc. Increasing the PRF, however, introduces a range ambiguity (see Chapter 7) that can raise some uncertainties about the real source of the echo signals.

Normally, a pulsed-Doppler transmitter sends out a burst of energy and counts time until echoes return from a specific region in the scanning plane. At that time, the receiver opens for a period equal to the transmit pulse length, then closes again (the range gate). The timing relationships for this situation are shown in Figure 8-22. Doubling the PRF creates a condition in which the receiver can accept echoes from two

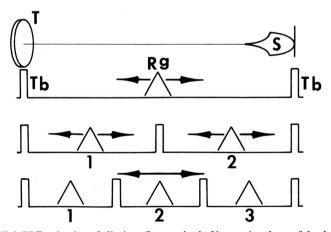

Figure 8-22   High PRF reduction of aliasing. One method of increasing the useful velocity range of a pulsed Doppler system is to increase the PRF. By doubling the maximum PRF for a maximum range, the system sees two range gates (*Rg*), one in the near half, the other in the far half of the range. Tripling the PRF produces three range gates, dividing the image range into thirds. *Tb* is the transmitting burst, *T* is the transducer, and *S* is the sample volume.

different locations. In other words, the number of range gates has increased to two. These two gates are separated by an interval equal to the pulse repetition interval. In addition, the signals are not all coming from the same pulse-listen cycle.

Unfortunately, the signals from the two sites add together in the tissue, preventing any easy separation of the two sources based on time alone. The separation of signal sites must come, instead, from the character of the signals. Often one sample volume is in stationary tissue while the other is in a cardiovascular compartment.

Elevating the PRF to three times normal increases the number of sample sites again (Fig. 8-22). Now the maximum range of the sonograph separates into three segments, with a range gate in each segment. All the sample sites move together, remaining always one-third the maximum distance apart. Each range gate handles a third of the whole field of view.

Each increase in PRF, of course, increases the maximum Doppler frequency the system can handle. The price paid for this increased capability is a decrease in the positional uniqueness of the sample volume. As the PRF increases, the number of sample sites increases at the same rate. At a theoretical limit of an infinite PRF is an infinite number of sample sites. And upon consideration, an infinite number of sample sites is really a CW Doppler with an infinite number of receiver range gates along the beam.

Unwrapping Signals

Another method of solving the aliasing problem is to unwrap the normal and aliased signals and reconstruct them.[9] This process reveals a new set of problems. It is equivalent to cutting the aliased signals and pasting them back on the top of the original waveform (Fig. 8-23). Essential to this analysis is an accurate determination of the aliasing signals. If the spectrum is noisy or has a large amount of spectral broadening, automatic unwrapping may not be possible. For very clean spectra with well-defined aliasing events, the correct signal output can be recreated by merging the aliased and unaliased portions of the output signal.

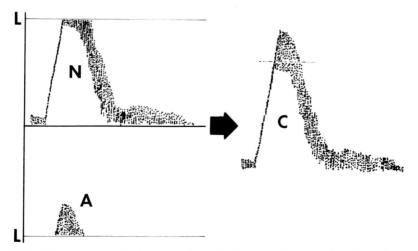

Figure 8-23   Unwrapping an aliasing spectral signal. One method of removing aliasing is to reconstruct the spectrum by placing the aliased segment (*A*) back on the normal segment (*N*), producing a complete spectrum (*C*). This is possible if no additional spectral broadening is present to hide the aliased segment. *L* represents the aliasing limits in each direction.

Moving the Input Signals

If increasing the PRF or changing the mathematics of analysis is not possible, then lowering the Doppler shift frequencies is an alternative. Moving from a 5.0-MHz to a 3.0-MHz operating frequency, for example, lowers all the Doppler shift frequencies, including the maximum frequency. The maximum signal may now be below the Nyquist limit.

Lowering the operating frequency, however, affects other aspects of the signal processing problem. First, a lower transmitting frequency reduces the reflection from blood.[4] Part of this reduction is offset, however, by a lower attenuation rate within tissues and a larger sample volume that can increase the average echo-signal energy. In addition, transducers with small diameters and lower frequencies do not focus as well as higher frequency transducers of the same size. The result is larger sample volumes, shorter effective focal zones, and more side lobes than with higher frequency transducers.

Lower Doppler shift frequencies can also come from a steeper Doppler angle. Moving to a more obtuse angle (approaching perpendicular to the blood movement) will reduce the Doppler shift frequencies. Often this is not possible because of the anatomy of the access window and the geometry of flow within a cardiovascular compartment. Flow within the heart is a good example of this sort of physical limitation. Here, blood flow is nearly parallel to the precordial cardiac window and perpendicular to the suprasternal and subcostal windows. Thus, flow is nearly perpendicular to the beam from the precordium but parallel to the beam from either the suprasternal or subcostal windows.

Lowering the frequency and increasing the Doppler angle decreases all the Doppler shift frequencies. Such a reduction includes some of the lower velocities that may be important to a diagnosis. This is more of a problem when looking at venous structures but vanishes when looking at the high velocities of the heart.

References

1. Barber, FE, Baker, DW, Nation, AWC, et al. Ultrasonic duplex echo-Doppler scanner. *IEEE Trans Biomed Eng* 21:109, 1974.
2. Pourcelot, L. Echo-Doppler systems applications for the detection of cardiovascular disorders. *In* Bom, N (ed): *Echocardiology With Doppler Applications and Real-Time Imaging.* The Hague: Martinus Nijhoff Medical, 1977, pp 245–256.
3. Baker, D, Lorch, G, and Rubinstein, S. Pulsed Doppler echocardiography. *In* Bom, N (ed): *Echocardiology With Doppler Applications and Real-Time Imaging.* The Hague: Martinus Nijhoff Medical, 1977, pp 207–222.
4. Atkinson, P, Woodcock, JP. *Doppler Ultrasound and Its Use in Clinical Measurement.* New York: Academic Press, 1982, pp 19, 37, 106.
5. McDicken, WN. *Diagnostic Ultrasonics Principles and Use of Instruments.* New York: John Wiley, 1981, p 62.
6. Baker, DW and Daigle, RE. Noninvasive ultrasound flowmetry. *In* Hwang, NHC and Normann, N (eds): *Cardiovascular Flow Dynamics and Measurements,* Baltimore: University Park Press, 1977, pp 151–189.
7. Powis, RL. Angiodynography: A new real time look at the vascular system. *Appl Radiol* 15:55–59, 1986.
8. Omoto, R (ed). *Color Atlas of Real-Time Two-Dimensional Doppler Echocardiology.* Tokyo: Shidan-To-Chiryo, 1984, p 11, 21.

9. Hatle, L, and Angelsen, B. *Doppler Ultrasound in Cardiology.* Philadelphia: Lea & Febiger, 1982, pp 51, 54, 211.
10. Ramirez, RW. *The FFT: Fundamentals and Concepts.* Beaverton, OR: Tektronix, Inc., 1975, pp 2–17.

9

Linking Doppler Displays with Physical Events

Setting a Course

Right now, the most widely used Doppler displays are Doppler sounds and spectral graphs. Doppler audio is the older of the two and carries a lot of raw information about flow events. Extracting enough details from Doppler sounds to draw clinical conclusions depends upon audio pattern recognition. It is a tough task, and most of this information remains hidden from the novice Doppler listener. It can even remain hidden from many of the more experienced users.

Spectral displays show the same sort of information, but unlike raw Doppler sounds, the information is processed for individual frequency components. The resulting graph has an unnatural form (for example, motion does not appear as arrows). Furthermore, the graph requires some reading skills to extract details about flow patterns. In the end, these reading skills center on a connection between the spectral display and the physical events within the vessels. The goal of this chapter is to forge the early links that eventually will help complete this connection.

Connecting the display and physical events is not so difficult now. Some excellent tools are available in the form of new color flow-imaging Doppler displays. These technologies provide an understandable depiction of blood flow patterns in two dimensions. Because these displays operate at or close to real time, the time course of the flow patterns is open to use as well. Color flow imaging will become a valuable link between physical flow events and the Doppler spectrum.

This discussion has several distinct parts. First, we consider the major events that occur in vessels and chambers of the heart. Second, we look for these events at the spectral display. Finally, to put some reality into the spectrum, we examine the capabilities and limitations inherent to a spectral display. We include the influences of the Doppler angle and the sample-volume geometry.

Major Flow Events

Using the spectral display as a tool begins with understanding the form of the information. The discussion then expands to include the central flow events.

Spectral Display Elements

A typical spectral display uses three axes of information as shown in Figure 9-1. On the vertical axis is frequency, expressed as discrete frequency bins if the Doppler analyzer is digital. It is nearly continuous if the Doppler signal analyzer is a zero crossing detector or a special analog design. For a fast Fourier transform (FFT) system, the frequency bins are distinct, discontinuous values. Each bin is a set of close frequencies that are treated as a single frequency and shown with a common gray-scale intensity.

Frequencies above the zero line represent forward flow, i.e., movement toward the transducer. Frequencies below the line represent reverse flow or motion away from the transducer.

The horizontal axis is time, which also progresses in distinct intervals if the output is from an FFT device. Each time step represents a sampling interval for the FFT, which may be as large as 300 ms or as small as 1 to 5 ms.

The third dimension in this display is the pixel gray scale. As the Fourier fre-

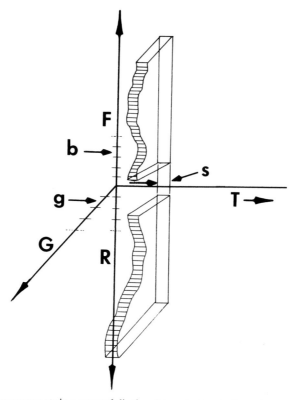

Figure 9-1 Basic components in a spectral display. At any instant in time, the spectral display shows a range of frequencies, forward (*F*) and reversed (*R*), with variable gray scale amplitudes (*G*), and these change over time (*T*). *b* is a frequency bin, *g* is the gray scale intensity, and *s* is the sampling interval.

quency components increase in strength, they appear with a predetermined gray-scale intensity, or in some displays, a specific color. As we learned from Chapter 7, a Fourier component amplitude (expressed as gray-scale intensity) is proportional to the number of red blood cells traveling in the same way to produce the same Doppler shift frequency.

Elements of Motion

An echo source moving at a constant velocity within an ultrasound field would produce a single Doppler frequency. A stationary echo source, on the other hand, produces a zero Doppler shift frequency. An accelerating echo source, however, produces a constantly increasing Doppler shift frequency if its *direction* of motion is unchanging. Clearly, a spectrum with signals moving away from the zero line represents accelerating echo sources, whereas signals moving toward the zero line represent decelerating echo sources.

Based on these simple ties between the spectral display and motion elements, the flow pattern from a normal vascular compartment marks out a definite sequence of events, which often begins with stationary red blood cells (as in the external carotid or femoral arteries). The sequence can also begin with slow moving blood, as in visceral arteries or the internal carotid artery, which have continuous flow throughout the cardiac cycle. As the pulse pressure reaches the cells within the ultrasound beam, they accelerate, causing an upward sweep in frequency (Fig. 9-2). As the driving energy reaches a maximum, blood motion also reaches a velocity maximum, which forms the peak of the waveform. As the pulse energy decreases, the blood decelerates, and the

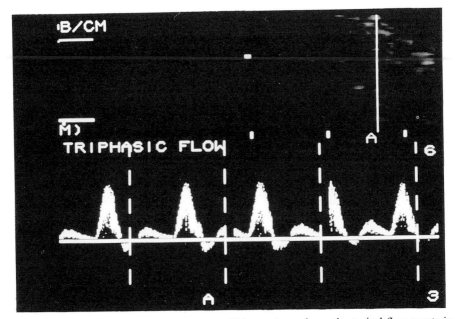

Figure 9-2 Typical vascular spectrum events. This spectrum shows the typical flow events in a lower limb artery (superficial femoral artery, [SFA]). Events begin with an acceleration phase containing a narrow range of frequencies. As the velocity reaches a peak, the flow gradients within the vessel slightly broaden the frequencies. Deceleration is more disorganized with broader frequencies. In this SFA waveform, a normal flow reversal occurs then forward flow again, forming a triphasic waveform. *A* is the spectral sampling cursor.

Doppler shift frequencies move toward zero. The events of accelerating, reaching a peak frequency, and decelerating, express the basic form of flow over time. And the shape of the signals over time represents physical events.

In general, during an acceleration phase, the driving pressure and the subsequent red blood cell motion are almost evenly distributed over the vessel lumen because of Pascal's law (Chapter 4). This common motion appears as a narrow spectral range as the blood accelerates. The narrowness clearly appears in a pulsed-Doppler output, but less so in a CW Doppler output that includes flow across the whole vessel. This blunt acceleration is a flow property found in vessels as well as chambers of the heart.

As motion progresses, however, the blood flow velocities distribute unevenly across the vessel lumen. The boundary layer, bound to the vessel wall surface and not moving, creates this uneven flow pattern. Thus, as motion increases in systole, the spectrum broadens.

The subsequent deceleration phase is affected by the fluid viscosity and velocity-dependent forces (Chapter 4). The uneven velocities leave an uneven momentum, and the slower portions of the flow decelerate first. As a result, blood movement is more disorganized during this period, which appears as a broadened spectrum.

Hydraulic Reflections

For many, it is a new thought to consider the pulse traveling through a vascular system as a wave. It is an approach that provides new analytical tools, predictions, and explanations for many observations of the vascular system.

Common to all waves is the ability to produce reflections where rapid changes in wave propagation properties occur.[1] In the vascular system, changes in the hydraulic impedance, i.e., changes in the ability to form hydraulic waves,[2] generate reflections. If the reflection is in phase with the incident wave, then as the two waves pass one another, they add to make the incident wave appear larger. An out-of-phase reflection, however, adds with the incident wave to decrease the apparent incident wave strength. The incident and reflected waves are, of course, traveling in different directions. The pressure at any point in the vessel is the sum of all the pressure waves traveling through that point at this time. This summing of hydraulic waves comes from the simple super-position properties of all waves.

Like ultrasound, the strength of a reflected hydraulic wave is proportional to the change in impedance seen by the incident wave.[3] At vessel bifurcations, the hydraulic impedance decreases. Reflections from the bifurcation are, thus, in phase with the incident wave. The pulse wave is a pressure wave, so pressure measurements just proximal to the bifurcation are slightly larger than pressures measured a little further upstream.[4] Measurements show a steadily increasing peak pulse pressure from the central vessels out to the periphery (Fig. 9-3). At the same time, the *average* pulse pressure is decreasing.

Between incident pulses, the hydraulic reflections travel back up the vessel, producing flow reversals in the whole vascular compartment. Figure 9-4 (see color section between pp. 116 and 117) shows an example of this reflection in a normal femoral artery. These reflections produce multiphasic flows with a net downstream component. Reflections of this sort make the flow pattern look as though the flow in the vessel were oscillating. Multiphasic flow patterns are not only normal, they are useful indicators of a normally changing hydraulic impedance.[5] The waveform changes as the peripheral vascular resistance changes.

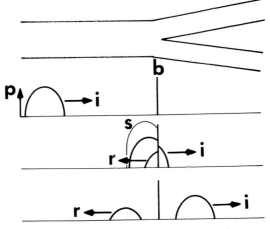

Figure 9-3 Pulse reflections at a change in hydraulic impedance in a vessel. The decrease in hydraulic impedance in a vessel causes an inphase reflection (*r*) of the incident pulse pressure (*p*) and adds to the incident pulse wave (*i*) near the vessel bifurcation (*b*). The result is an increasing pulse pressure (*s*) as the pulse travels more peripherally in the vascular system.

Hydraulic reflections can theoretically occur anytime during the cardiac cycle. According to angiodynographic findings and other, more invasive measures, they are usually present in late systole and early diastole. A downstream, femoral artery stenosis, for example, can make a normally triphasic-flow waveform both high amplitude and monophasic. In contrast, an upstream stenosis produces a low-amplitude, monophasic waveform. The first comes from hydraulic reflections, the second from damping the incident wave[5] (Fig. 9-5, see color section between pp. 116 and 117).

Laminar Flow

Stable flow through a straight vessel is usually laminar, with layers of fluid slipping over one another. Typically, the highest velocity is in the center of the lumen, with decreasing values toward the walls (Fig. 9-6). Finally, at the walls is a boundary layer of stationary fluid in direct contact with the wall.

Parabolic, laminar flow normally occurs under steady-state conditions when the driving energy is constant. In the vascular system, however, the cardiac cycle constantly changes the flow pattern. Very early in systole, the pulse pressure (potential energy) distributes evenly across the vessel lumen. This forms a blunt velocity profile across the vessel lumen as the blood accelerates. The boundary layer does not move, however. Blood movement, then, becomes uneven as the blood's internal resistance (viscosity) causes a flow velocity gradient to form. This gradient extends from the lumen's central axis out to the walls (Fig. 9-6).

The lower velocities near the wall show up in a spectrum as a duplex sample volume approaches the vessel walls. If the sample volume should include the wall, then a strong, low-frequency signal may swamp some of the more subtle aspects of the blood flow, especially the low-velocity signals from close to the boundary or stationary layer.

In general, a laminar flow pattern shows a nearly even distribution of Fourier component amplitudes.[6] Over the cardiac cycle, the narrowest frequency range appears during early systole.[6]

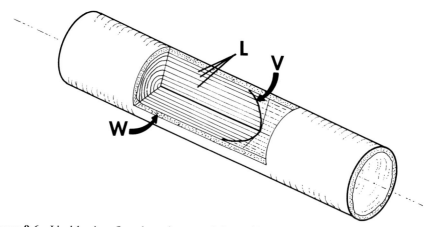

Figure 9-6   Ideal laminar flow through a vessel. In an ideal system, wetting the walls (*W*) of the vessel forms the boundary layer, which causes the formation of a parabolic velocity (*V*) distribution over the vessel diameter. *L* represents the small layers (lamellae) of fluid motion.

Vessel Narrowing

As blood approaches a vessel narrowing, flow velocities increase. This acceleration increases the Doppler shift frequencies while changing the Fourier component amplitudes. The acceleration makes the velocity profile blunter, and at the same time, the difference between the blunt flow and the boundary layer is greater. The frequency content is larger, with higher frequencies representing higher velocities. Figure 9-7 shows this relationship.

Within a 70% narrowing, the laminar flow pattern vanishes. If the velocities are high enough, fluid flow stability is lost, and high-velocity eddies can form within the blood moving near the lumen walls.[7] The high velocities and loss of flow organization cause elevated spectral frequencies and spectral broadening (Fig. 9-7).

If the poststenotic lumen opens up rapidly, the flowing blood cannot respond fast enough to fill it with streamlines. Many small flow separations and poststenotic tur-

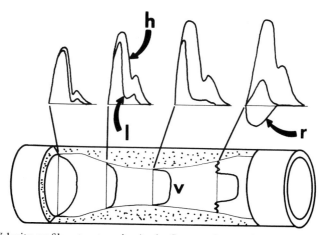

Figure 9-7   Velocity profiles at a stenosis. As the flow accelerates through a stenosis, the spectral frequencies increase and broaden (*l* is the lowest frequency, *h* is the highest). *v* is the velocity profile. At the distal end of the stenosis, flow reversals, separations, vortices, and eddy currents can occur (*r*) near the edge of the flow pattern.

bulence are the result (Fig. 9-7). The separations are a consequence of the rapidly expanding vessel lumen; the turbulence comes from the fluid instabilities. They combine to produce the poststenotic events.

Turbulence

As the flow velocities push beyond the bounds of stable flow at the outlet of a stenosis, the streamlines break up and movement becomes chaotic. Eddies and small vortices form and travel downstream with the bulk flow in the fluid.[8] Within the turbulent region, the velocities may be very high, with a great deal of spectral broadening (Fig. 9-7). Farther downstream, the expanding lumen creates an even greater range of velocities and Doppler frequencies. As a result, the spectrum becomes very broad. This is where we look to detect and evaluate vascular disease with a Doppler system.[9]

Turbulence produces a loss of the normal pressure-flow relationship. Normally, increasing the driving pressure increases the volume flow proportionately. In the face of turbulence, this is no longer the case. Now, as the driving pressure increases, the energy contributing *to the turbulence* increases. Because this additional energy goes only into the chaotic behavior, volume flow remains nearly constant.[10] These changes are shown in Figure 9-8. Indeed, increasing the driving pressure merely makes the flow more chaotic without increasing the volume flow.

Poststenotic turbulence (Fig. 9-7) expends energy largely in the form of heat, as the vortices and eddies work against the blood viscosity. Part of the energy can go into the mechanical vibration of the vessel walls and surrounding tissues (a bruit). As eddy currents and vortices expend energy, they die out, and the flow pattern eventually regains its stable, laminar quality. How far this disturbance extends downstream is in some respects a measure of the severity of the stenosis. In general, however, how fast the blood moves in systole (peak systolic frequencies) and the amount of flow disorganization (spectral broadening) are better measures of stenosis.[11]

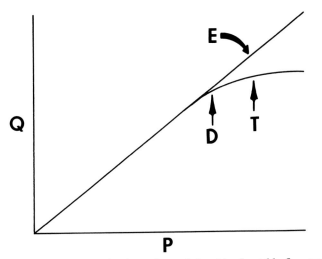

Figure 9-8   The driving pressure and volume flow relationship. In stable flow patterns, a linear relationship exists between the driving pressure (*P*) and the volume flow rate (*Q*). As instabilities develop in the flow, an increase in pressure does not increase the flow rate in the same manner (*D*). Finally, at full turbulence (*T*), an increasing pressure produces no increase in volume flow rate. *E* is the expected stable flow rate.

Flow Separations

Even if a flow process is essentially stable and laminar, flow separations will occur when the vessel wall moves out from the flow faster than the fluid streamlines can follow. Flow separations can also occur when wall irregularities direct the streamlines away from the wall for a short distance. Along with lumen expansions, vessel tortuosities create geometric changes that blood can not follow.[8] As the fluid flow pattern detaches from the vessel wall, a separation bubble appears that creates an oversized boundary layer. During systole, these separation bubbles contain reversed or circular flow. During diastole, movement in the bubble is much slower than the stream of blood passing nearby. Flow may even be stagnant over portions of diastole. The geometry of a flow separation is shown in Figure 9-9.

Blood flow within a separation bubble comes from the difference in pressure that exists between the rapidly moving blood in the major streamline and the stationary blood in the bubble. The Venturi effect lowers the pressure in the moving blood (predicted by the Bernoulli equation) while the separation bubble has a higher pressure. As a result, the blood reverses through the separation bubble, flowing toward the lower pressure streamline. An example of a large flow separation appears in Figure 9-10 (see color section between pp. 116 and 117).

Detecting a separation process in a vessel requires both a sample volume and spatial sampling smaller than the separation layer. Large sample volumes combine the forward and reversed flow together at the separation boundary. This creates a Doppler shift waveform that looks more turbulent than just disturbed. And in truth, a flow separation is much more organized than shown in a single spectral recording. Figures 9-10 and 9-11 (see color section) show some of the flow patterns and waveforms commonly found in the carotid artery bulb of normal people. They look disturbed and typically add a warbling quality to the Doppler sounds.

If a lumen slowly and smoothly decreases, the result can be a narrowing that forms neither separations nor turbulence. These vessels show only elevated frequencies and moderate spectral broadening. Figure 9-12 (see color section) shows how an angiodynogram depicts such a gradual, smooth vessel narrowing.

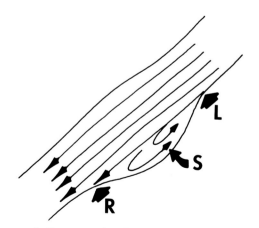

Figure 9-9   The geometry of a flow separation. In a flow separation, the streamlines leave the wall (*L*) and reconnect (*R*), producing a separation bubble (*S*) containing flow reversals and turbulence in systole. This occurs in flow geometries in which the walls change direction faster than the flow can follow.

Turbulence is a major disruption of the streamlines, producing spectral broadening. Flow separations can also contribute significantly to any spectral broadening. Indeed, flow separations form the eddies and vortices characteristic of turbulent flow. Large sample volumes and spectral analysis alone will fall short in separating complex, yet stable, flow patterns from true turbulence. Large sample volumes combine too much flow, and a single-point spectrum cannot show the flow in the vicinity of the sample volume.

Blunt Flow

Blunt flow occurs under two basic conditions: first, in early systole, when the driving pressure first appears and acceleration is nearly uniform; second, when flow enters a pipe from a much larger reservoir. The first condition is common during early systole in nearly all vessels, but the bluntness soon disappears as blood moves and fluid viscosity forms velocity gradients. The pulmonary artery and aorta, however, represent an unusually stable situation in which the velocity profile is blunt over a large part if not all of the cardiac ejection cycle. This reliable blunt flow pattern in the aorta, for example, makes CW and pulsed-Doppler estimates of cardiac output possible without having to map velocity profiles.

As blood enters a vessel narrowing, a blunt flow pattern forms from both an entry effect (movement from a larger to a smaller orifice) and an acceleration from the arriving pulse pressure.

Wall Roughening

Rough spots on the walls of a pipe can create small local eddy currents and vortices that indicate the presence of these rougheniings.[8] The same is true within the vascular system. In general, wall irregularities must extend into the lumen some distance greater than the boundary layer thickness to disturb the flow pattern. Thus, when flow is laminar and streamlines are close to the wall, an irregularity need not be very large to generate a disturbance. In contrast, a wall irregularity in a flow separation must be physically large to break up the primary flow pattern or the flow reversal through a separation bubble. Some rough-wall eddy currents are shown in Figure 9-13 (see color section).

Along with size, a disturbing wall irregularity also needs to have the right shape. For example, a plaque with a smooth surface may not break up streamlines, and flow over the surface will be both laminar and undisturbed. If the trailing edge of a plaque is sharp, however, the edge can generate a series of vortices that travel downstream for a short distance.

Rough-wall disturbances are hard to see in a conventional duplex system because close to the wall, the disturbance and wall movement are summed into the same echo-signal. Angiodynography, however, has a spatial image resolution that is small enough to show the patterns of flow associated with vessel wall roughening.

Ventricular Filling

Mechanical models and color flow imaging in the left ventricle show a rather complex filling sequence.[12] Blood does not simply pour into the ventricle from the left atrium; instead, it forms a large vortex. The vortex center begins to form as atrial blood moves toward the apex of the heart through the mitral valve as an organized fluid column. The flowing blood then sweeps up the walls of the ventricle from apex to base, as shown in Figure 9-14. The flowing blood then turns again near the base of the heart to blend in with the blood still flowing from the left atrium.

This filling sequence is clear in both the M-mode and real-time imaging of the mitral valve. An M-mode recording of the two mitral valve leaflets first shows separation as the valve opens to form the early passive filling phase. As the filling vortex forms and blood sweeps up the ventricular walls, the mitral valve leaflets move toward one another, completing the passive filling phase. When the left atrium contracts, the active portion of ventricular filling begins, separating the leaflets once more. The leaflets then close again as the vortex moves behind them. These events are quite visible in Figure 9-15. Mitral valve closure finally occurs as the ventricle contracts, building the intra-ventricular pressure.

If the heart rate is slow, passive filling can show several rotations of the vortex. When this happens, valve motion becomes a series of anterior valve leaflet movements quite like the first part of passive filling, and the valve appears to oscillate (Fig. 9-16).

Within the left ventricular inflow tract, the filling sequence is passive and then active. The result is an M-shaped flow sequence that looks a lot like the M-mode recording of the mitral valve. Figure 9-17 shows the spectrum of left ventricular filling.

Ventricular Emptying

Acceleration and entry processes govern events in the ejection of blood into the aorta. A sample volume in a ventricular streamline that passes through the aortic orifice produces a spectrum that looks like an ascending aorta waveform. An example of a left ventricular outflow wave form is shown in Figure 9-18.

During ejection, the heart contracts in a symmetrical manner, but the heart's

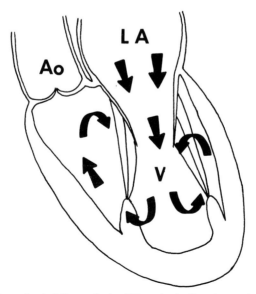

Figure 9-14   Vortex formation in left ventricular filling. As the flow (*arrows*) enters the left ventricle (*V*) from the left atrium (*LA*), the flow pattern circles behind the mitral valve leaflets, passively closing them during the filling process. *Ao* is the aorta.

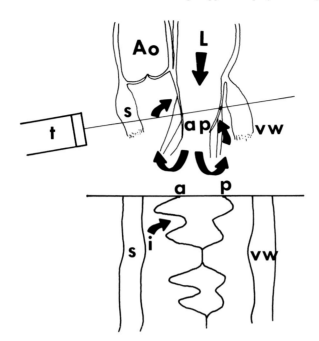

Figure 9-15   Passive closing of mitral leaflets with ventricular filling. M-mode recording in the lower half of the figure tracks the motion of the left ventricle walls and valve leaflets. *a* and *p* mark the anterior and posterior leaflets of the mitral valve in both the anatomical drawing and lower recording. *i* marks the passive closure of the valve. *L* is the left atrium, *vw* is the ventricular wall, *s* is the septum, *Ao* is the aorta, and *t* is the transducer.

movement is opposite to the moving blood.[13] Thus, as blood moves out the left ventricular outflow tract, the heart reacts to the ejection by moving downward. This reaction to blood ejection is the same sort as propels jet aircraft and rockets. The downward motion stores a portion of the ejection energy in the elastic qualities of the great vessels and the myocardium. From the point of view of the heart, the blood velocity and the downward heart movement combine to create a *relative* blood velocity higher than we can measure with Doppler from outside the body.

At the end of ejection, the heart relaxes and moves upward toward the great vessels. This carries the remaining blood in the outflow tract with it. During this period, aortic regurgitation from incompetent valves is visible. Mapping the penetration of the jet into the ventricular cavity can estimate the severity of the valve incompetence.[14]

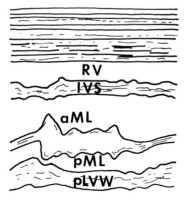

Figure 9-16   Multiple leaflet motion of the mitral valve. A relatively slow heart rate can often show mitral valve leaflet oscillations (*aVL* and *pVL*) as vortex filling occurs. *RV* is the right ventricle, *IVS* is the interventricular septum, and *pLVW* is the posterior, left ventricular wall.

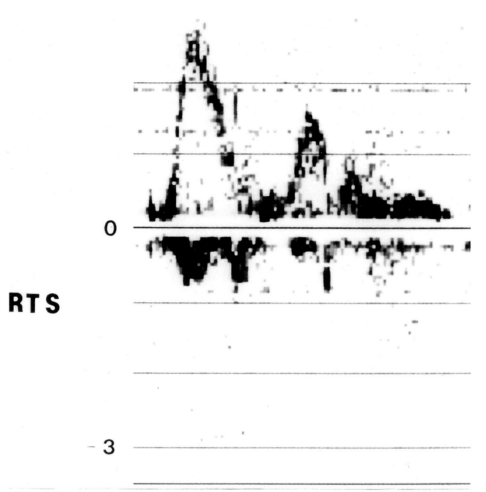

Figure 9-17   Flow in the left ventricle through the mitral valve. The active and passive flow events through the mitral valve fill the left ventricle. The first portion of the flow is passive, the second pulse is active atrial contraction. The result is an M shape very like the M-mode motion pattern of the mitral valve.

Limitations in Doppler Signal Processing

Failing to understand the inherent limitations in Doppler signal processing opens the door to easy misinterpretations of the spectral results that could be professionally embarrassing.

Sample Volume Accuracy

A primary assumption in duplex imaging is that the sample volume location on the display is the same as in the tissue. All too often, the real location is something different from what is on the screen. And of all the parameters of a duplex sonograph that can drift, this is one of the easiest to measure. A *normal* vessel or a simple test object made of a string moving over a pulley in water are sufficient to test the accuracy of the range gate location. Figure 9-19 shows how to use a string test object.

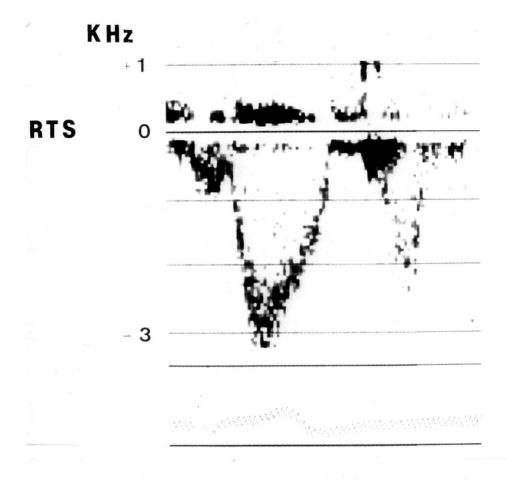

K Hz

+ 1

RTS   0

– 3

Figure 9-18 Flow through the left ventricular outflow tract. In this example, the left ventricular flow is recorded from a subcostal view, sampling below the initial valve. Flow is away from the transducer (reversed) and shaped like flow within the ascending aorta.

Of course, a Doppler phantom can also test the ultrasound system for positional accuracy as well as other parameters. A Doppler phantom differs from the string test object, however. A phantom is typically made of tissue-mimicking material with attenuation and scattering sites distributed through the medium. Synthetic blood moves through simulated vessels in the phantom, driven by an external pump. Along with a test for range-gate axial position accuracy should also be a test for lateral position accuracy inside the image scanning plane.

Accurately positioning a receiver range gate depends on the accuracy of the internal 13-μs clock. This clock provides the 1-cm range intervals and depth markers. Measuring the range-gate position depends on the ability to count time accurately from the start of transmission for each pulse-listen cycle. Lateral position accuracy depends upon knowing where the Doppler beam points in space, and that can become complicated. Whatever the source of the error, inaccurate sampling can give zero flow for a normal vessel, or an acceptable flow from a normal adjacent vessel instead of the vessel under investigation. These problems expand geometrically, especially if the vessel and sample volume are very small and a long distance from the Doppler transducer.

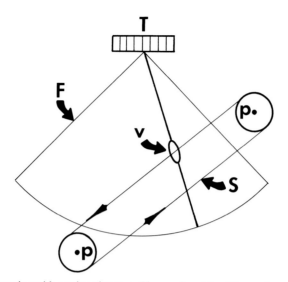

Figure 9-19   Basic testing with a string phantom. The moving string (*S*), passing over pulleys (*p*), in the phantom represents a calibrated moving echo source. It can test not only Doppler processing but positioning of the sample volume (*v*) within the scanning field (*F*). *T* is the transducer array.

If the Doppler beam and image beam are the same, then sample volume position remains automatically in the scanning plane. If the Doppler beam is from an outboard transducer, then positioning must also keep the Doppler beam inside the image-scanning plane.

A Real View of the Spectrum

Because Doppler signal processing is so poorly understood, it is easy to look at a spectral output and equate this display with the Doppler sounds. Putting an oscilloscope on the audio output from a Doppler system can quickly dispel this notion. Figure 9-20 shows an example of an unprocessed Doppler signal waveform.

The Doppler sounds are the superposition of many individual signals. These waves add together to form the final shape in the oscilloscope (Fig. 9-20). It is a situation where the frequencies make the shape of the wave, and altering the shape of the wave changes the frequencies the wave contains. In essence, the frequency content of the signal and shape of the signal mean the same thing. As a result, frequencies found in spectral analysis can be changed by anything that changes the shape of the composite audio signal. The spectral output from a Doppler system is a processed output. Any distortions to the signal shape on the way to the processing can take away or add Fourier frequency components to the final spectrum. Nonlinear amplifiers in the Doppler signal stream and very small sample volumes contribute to this sort of Doppler signal modulation and misreading of the spectrum.

A clue to the presence and severity of vascular disease is spectral broadening, which is a measure of flow organization. The greater the disorganization, the greater the number of frequencies present in the spectrum. Disorganization, of course, is an indication of disease, and thus the link between disease and spectral broadening. Disease, however, is not the only way of producing spectral broadening in a Doppler output.

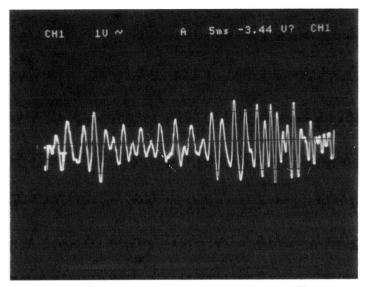

Figure 9-20 Raw Doppler signals from a normal common carotid artery. The unprocessed Doppler signal is the sum of all the waves that are present. This complex waveform shows two cardiac cycles from a normal common carotid artery.

The first way of creating broadening is to modulate the shape of the Doppler signal (Figure 9-21, A). This modulation occurs when blood moves through a very narrow sample volume (tightly focused beam) very fast.[15] The thin ultrasound beam shortens and steepens the Doppler signal. This change in shape is the same as adding large-amplitude, higher frequency waves. The narrower and steeper the Doppler signals, the higher the frequencies that contribute to that shape, increasing spectral content.

Spectral broadening can also occur when a large sample volume sits in a steep velocity gradient (Figure 9-21, B). This can happen when larger sample volumes include a significant portion of a complex flow pattern within a vessel. For example, turning vessels can push major streamlines near a wall, making the velocity change very quickly from the wall to the central streamline. Any asymmetric velocity profile can look broadened if the range gate is sitting on the edge of the flow pattern.

Flow that turns within a sample volume is another way of producing a broad range of spectral frequencies (Fig. 9-21, C). Looking into the transverse aorta with a large sample volume often produces spectral broadening as the blood flow turns within the large sample volume. Flow around the corner of a kinked or tortuous vessel is an excellent source of spectral broadening without stenosis.

Another source of spectral broadening is the chaotic behavior of fluids. In this pattern, the streamlines are broken and disturbed, but the vessel does not have obstructive disease (Fig. 9-21, D). The source of this flow behavior is unclear, but it is a well-established phenomenon in hydrodynamics. It is also visible in angiodynograms as a mottling of the color, representing the breakup of streamlines. The spectrum from this flow pattern shows broadening without the acceleration characteristic of stenosis (Fig. 9-22, see color section between pp. 116 and 117).

Of course, the obvious source of spectral broadening is obstructive disease that breaks up the normal vascular flow pattern (Fig. 9-21, E). It requires some reading skill to make sure that spectral broadening is truly from disease and not from some other, nonpathological source.

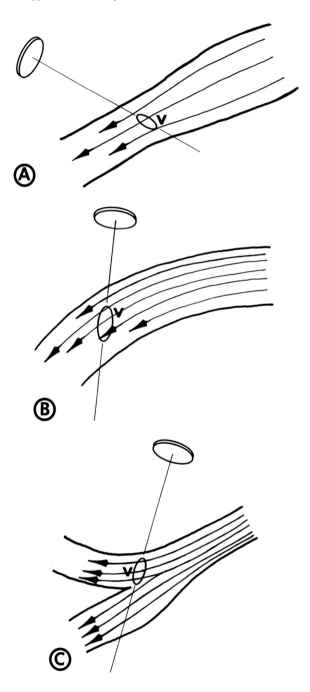

Figure 9-21.   A–C   Sources of spectral broadening in normal blood flow. **A,** A small sample volume (*v*) and a high velocity can modulate the signals, creating additional frequencies. **B,** A sample volume (*v*) sitting at the edge of a flow velocity gradient will produce spectral broadening. **C,** A sample volume (*v*) in a turning streamline will produce spectral broadening. **D,** A sample volume (*v*) within in-line turbulence will produce spectral broadening. **E,** All these events occur in the poststenotic pattern. *J* is the jet, *g* is flow gradient, *t* is turbulence, and *h* is high velocity flow.

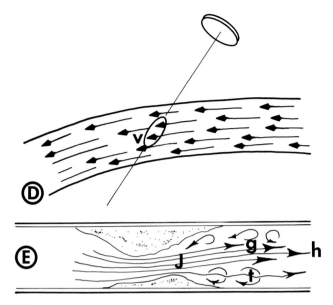

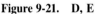

Figure 9-21. D, E

Flow Pattern Assumptions

Because we cannot easily see the two-dimensional flow pattern in a cardiovascular compartment by using duplex imaging only, some traditional assumptions guide our conclusions. Unfortunately, several of these assumptions are only sometimes true.

    Two traditional assumptions about flow in a vascular compartment are that the maximum velocity is in the center of the vessel and that the velocity profile centers on the vessel axis. In reality, flow is seldom down the middle and parallel to the walls, unless the flow meets some strict physical conditions. First, the flow must be laminar and *undisturbed*. Second, the vessel must be physically straight for a significant portion of its length. In the real world, however, vessels curve in space. At the same time, blood has both mass and momentum so that, as vessels turn, higher velocity portions of the flow veer away from the vessel axis in a turning vessel. If vessels happen to be tortuous enough, an undisturbed flow pattern becomes physically impossible, and the axial flow pattern assumption does not hold true. That means, to define accurately what is happening, we need to know more about the real flow pattern.

    The next major assumption is that a stenotic vessel or valve produces a jet that is axial to the vessel or valve. At the outset, stenotic diseases that develop from an expanding plaque are seldom really symmetrical.[16] As a consequence, jets from stenosis can aim in virtually any direction within a vascular compartment. These off-axis jets are an excellent opportunity to overcall or undercall the severity of disease (Fig. 9-23). Figure 9-24 shows the problems of measuring Doppler frequencies in a deviated jet. Nonsymmetrical jets can also occur in the heart. Calculating a pressure gradient by estimating a jet velocity can be problematic when the jet moves way from its expected central axis (Fig. 9-24).

    What makes these jet deviations so uncomfortable is that they are invisible to the single-point duplex system. A duplex device has no inherent way of determining flow

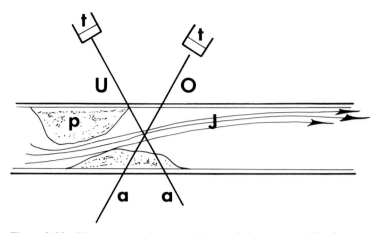

Figure 9-23   The geometry of a non-axial stenotic jet. A nonaxial jet formation can create problems in estimating Doppler frequencies. Looking upstream at this jet (*J*) will overestimate (*O*) the frequencies. Looking downstream will underestimate (*U*) the frequencies. *t* is the transducer, *a* is the
beam axis, and *p* is the vessel plaque.

direction other than toward or away from the transducer. And without very careful,
time-consuming, detailed sampling coupled with some insights on the way blood flows,
a user has little chance of detecting these deviations. Color flow imaging and angiodynography, however, automatically carry out the detailed sampling needed to depict
flow deviations.

Flow Angle and Spectral Content

The spectral content of a flow signal changes with a changing Doppler angle.[17] For
example, as the Doppler angle approaches zero (parallel to the flow), the Doppler shift
frequencies become higher and broader. This results from the increasing difference
between the very low boundary layer frequencies and the maximum velocity frequency. At the same time, the blood takes more time to traverse the ultrasound beam,

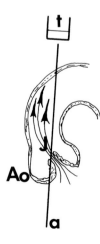

Figure 9-24   The geometry of a nonaxial aortic jet. Estimates of distal aortic
stenosis jets (*J*) can be in error if the jet is not axial to the lumen. In this
geometry, a jet thought to be axial is nearly 45° to the ultrasound beam. *Ao* is
the aorta, *t* is the transducer, and *a* is the beam axis.

reducing some of the amplitude modulation effects. Because the maximum frequency and the range of frequencies in a spectrum depend upon the Doppler angle, accurate frequency estimates need a constant Doppler angle. And a known Doppler angle is central to any velocity calculations. A common value used for the vascular system is 60°.[17]

A rather insidious Doppler angle error can occur, however, when a thick Doppler ultrasound beam hides the true Doppler angle in the image. It is easy to think of a beam as a two-dimensional object when it is really three-dimensional. A flow pattern that spirals within the scanning plane but does not appear to turn in the two-dimensional projection can create both unexpected spectral broadening and errors in estimating flow velocities. It is not good enough to work out flow patterns in only two dimensions when trying to estimate flow velocities accurately. That third dimension must be checked. Again, working out the flow patterns with duplex is very time consuming but is both easier and much faster with color flow imaging.

Changing Sample Volume Geometry

Spectral frequency content is clearly a function of the flow pattern but not so clearly a function of the sample volume size and shape. Large and small sample volumes within the same flow, for example, will not contain the same range of frequencies because they do not include the same portion of the flow events.

The lateral size of a sample volume depends upon the effectiveness of the beam geometry. In an electronically focused transducer, the beam geometry may be nearly the same over a large part of the image. Mechanically focused transducers, however, have a constantly changing beam. It is wide close to the transducer, narrow in the focal zone, and wide again beyond the focal zone. Clearly, the Doppler sample volume width for a fixed-focus transducer is going to vary along the beam. Any mechanically focused transducer will have a region of best performance that corresponds to the focal zone. Within the focal zone, the steady beam formation offers the most consistent sample volume geometry. Clearly, the best place to compare the spectra among different patients and events is within the focal zone.

Transducers that use phasing techniques electronically focus on transmitting and receiving cycles. These transducers include the linear arrays, phased arrays, and annular arrays. By making the focusing dynamic, these transducers can produce a nearly constant sample volume geometry over a large portion of the image.[19] Many of the linear arrays permit combining a lot of transducer elements to make larger transducing apertures. As a result, these transducers often have better focusing control over longer distances than smaller linear phased arrays.

The larger linear arrays and the smaller linear phased arrays have a common focusing problem. Focusing along the array is both electronic and relatively good. Transverse to the arrays, however, the focusing is not electronic. Focusing in this direction typically comes from a cylindrical lens that creates a fixed focal point with a long focal zone. The result is an asymmetric sample volume architecture with strong focusing along the array and limited, fixed focusing transverse to the array. In general, the dynamic focusing along the array minimizes the effects from the mechanical focusing. Figure 9-25A shows the formation of these two types of focusing for the linear array.

A phased array that avoids this transverse focusing problem is the annular array (Fig. 9-25, B). Instead of having the transducer elements in a line, this array has ele-

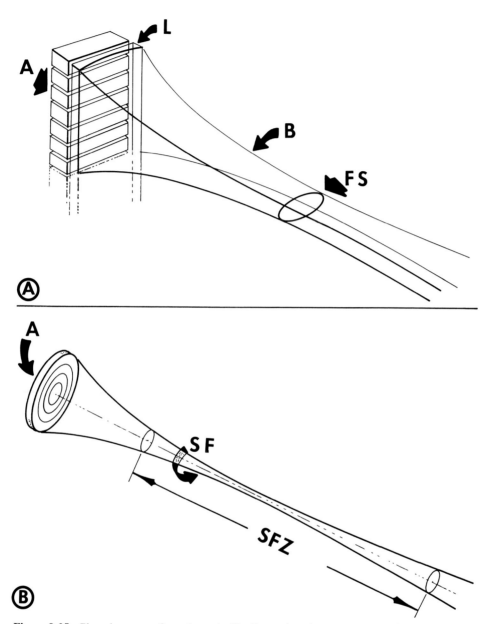

Figure 9-25   Phased array configurations. **A,** The linear phased array uses a set of linear elements (*A*) that electronically form a beam (*B*), with an asymmetric focal spot (*FS*). In general, a linear phased array is small, with more than 64 elements, whereas a phased linear array is larger with up to 500 elements. Focusing transverse to the array comes from a mechanical lens (*L*). **B,** The phased annular array uses circular elements (*A*) to form a symmetrically focused beam (*SF*). Dynamic focusing can provide very long, narrow focal zones (*SFZ*).

ments shaped into concentric rings. Like a single-element, circular transducer, the annular array can hold a sample volume geometry that is symmetrical about the beam axis. The individual transducing elements, however, permit variable focusing techniques, producing a beam width that can be nearly constant over very long distances.

References

1. Edmonds, PD, and Dunn, F: Introduction. Physical Description of Ultrasonic Fields. *In* Edmonds, PD (ed): *Methods of Experimental Physics: Ultrasonics*. New York: Academic Press, 1981, pp 1–28.
2. Bergel, DH: Blood flow dynamics. *In* Perronneau, P and Diebold, B (eds): *Cardiovascular Applications of Doppler Echography*. Publication 111. Paris: Institut National de la Santé et de la Recherche Medicale publication, 1982, pp 65–80.
3. Dinnar, U. *Cardiovascular Fluid Dynamics*. Boca Raton: CRC Press, 1981, p 95.
4. Jensen, D. *The Principles of Physiology*. New York: Appleton-Century-Crofts. 1976, p 636.
5. Johnston, KW, Maruzzo, BC, Kassam, M, et al. Methods for obtaining, processing and quantifying Doppler blood velocity waveforms. *In* Nicolaides, AN and Yao, JST (eds): *Investigation of Vascular Disorders*. New York: Churchill Livingston, 1981, pp 532–558.
6. Peronneau, P, Herment, A, Moutet, J, et al. Analyse Du Signal Doppler. *In* Perronneau, P and Diebold, B (eds): *Cardiovascular Applications of Doppler Echography*. Publication 111. Paris: Institut National de la Santé et de la Recherche Medicale publication, 1982, pp 81–114.
7. Rittgers, SE, Putney, WW, and Barnes, RW. Early detection of stroke-related lesions by real-time Doppler spectral analysis. *In* Hershey, FB, Barnes, RW, and Sumner, DS (eds): *Noninvasive Diagnosis of Vascular Disease*. Pasadena, CA: Appleton-Davies, 1984, pp 248–257.
8. Rouse, H. *Elementary Mechanics of Fluids*. New York: Dover Publications, 1946, pp 25–27, 195, 248.
9. Roederer, GO, Langlois, Y, and Strandness, DE Jr. Comprehensive noninvasive evaluation of extracranial cerebrovascular disease. *In* Hershey, FB, Barnes, RW, and Sumner, D (eds): *Noninvasive Diagnosis of Vascular Disease*. Pasadena, California: Appleton Davies, Inc., 1984, pp 177–216.
10. Burton, AC. *Physiology and Biophysics of the Circulation*. Chicago: Year Book Medical, 1965, p 134.
11. Keagy, BA, Pharr, WF, Thomas, D, et al. Objective criteria for the interpretation of carotid artery spectral analysis patterns. *Angiology* 33:213–220, 1982.
12. Bellhouse, B, and Williams, W. From Left Atrium to Left Ventricle. *In* Perronneau, P and Diebold, B (eds): *Cardiovascular Applications of Doppler Echography*. Publication 111. Paris: Institut National de la Santé et de la Recherche Medicale publication, 1982, pp 411–426.
13. Robinson, TF, Factor, SM, and Sonnenblick, EH. The heart as a suction pump. *Sci Am* 254:84–91, 1986.
14. Ciobanu, M, Abassi, AS, Allen, M, et al. Pulsed Doppler echocardiography in the diagnosis and estimation of severity of aortic insufficiency. *Am J Cardiol* 49:339–343, 1982.
15. Baker, DW and Daigle, RE. Noninvasive ultrasonic flowmetry. *In* Hwang, NHC and Normann, NA (eds): *Cardiovascular Flow Dynamics and Measurements*. Baltimore: University Park Press, 1977, pp 151–189.
16. Hennerici, M, Reiffschneider, G, and Sandmann, W. Detection of early atherosclerotic lesions from duplex-scanning of the carotid artery. *In* Perronneau, P and Diebold, B (eds): *Cardiovascular Applications of Doppler Echography*. Publication 111. Paris: Institut National de la Santé et de la Recherche Medicale publication, 1982, pp 191–198.
17. Gill, RW. Measurement of blood flow by ultrasound: Accuracy and sources of error. *Ultrasound Med Biol* 11:625–641, 1985.
18. Somer, JC. Phased array systems. *In* Bom, N. (ed) *Echocardiology with Doppler Applications and Real Time Imaging*. The Hague: Martinus Nijhoff Medical, 1977, pp 325–334.

10

Quantitation and Doppler Ultrasound

Quantitation Overview

The switch from listening to Doppler sounds to estimating the discrete Fourier components of a Doppler signal is a move from qualitative to quantitative Doppler analysis. At the heart of this move is the fast Fourier transform (FFT) device. All of the quantitative steps we use today depend on an accurate estimate of one or more of the Doppler signal frequency components. In addition, we need an accurate depiction of how they change over time.

This shift in emphasis is more than just the fallout from a new technology; it is the consequence of a new attitude toward Doppler ultrasound and its role in diagnostics. This change in attitude seems to have started in Europe, culminating in the Doppler-based quantitative tools for evaluating the heart as a pump.[1]

Doppler quantitation really has two aspects. First is the mathematical estimate of the Fourier frequency components. This step eclipsed the use of audio analysis and the zero-crossing detector as analytical tools. The second aspect is the use of Fourier frequency components to calculate other parameters that help us detect and evaluate disease in the heart and vascular system.

Because the perceived value of quantitation is growing, an FFT analysis is only the first step. Current displays not only show the Doppler spectrum of Fourier frequency components but also parameters such as the maximum, minimum, mean, and mode frequencies. Often additional statistics or calculations are available to the user, all based on the original estimates of these Fourier components.

In this chapter we look at some of the current quantitative techniques that use Doppler signals and spectra. Along with these tools, however, comes a requirement to understand the limitations of the calculations. Numbers intrinsically carry no information about how they were formed, and it is easy to place too much reliance on a number that is in reality based on a very shaky assumption. Numbers seem believable because they are numbers, derived from the rigorous rules of arithmetic that we all believe. In the end, we may not doubt the arithmetic, but testing the assumptions behind the arithmetic may be very valuable.

Making calculations requires controlling several machine and Doppler-dependent variables, including such things as Doppler angle, system output power, signal processing gain, and gray scale assignment. The price of objectivity is a more critical look at the physical and electronic events that surround Doppler calculations.

Complicating all Doppler calculations is the normal biological variability of the human in health and disease. Values for physiological parameters must always be couched in the context of the individual and other indications of vascular function.

Quantitation and Fluid Behavior

Quantitation requires some assumptions about how fluids behave, and in particular, how blood behaves. These can be summed into a few simple rules that weave through the various mathematics:

1. Pressure is applied equally in all directions. As we learned from Chapter 4, this also means that pressure does not propagate through a fluid instantly but at the acoustic propagation velocity. It also means that a vascular pressure wave is initially felt uniformly across a vessel lumen. As movement occurs, the boundary layer establishes a velocity gradient across the lumen.
2. Predicting flow requires accounting for all forms of energy associated with a moving fluid. This energy sum is the Bernoulli equation, which includes kinetic energy, gravitational energy, inertial work on the blood, and velocity-dependent resistance.
3. In general, fluid mass is neither made nor destroyed; therefore, the amount of blood entering a vessel must be equal to the amount leaving that vessel. In a simple sense, this is the conservation of mass: what goes in must come out.
4. Blood flow is always down an energy gradient, not just a pressure gradient. Thus, pressure can change temporally and spatially, but flow continues down the energy gradient. In some instances, the driving pressure can be opposite to the flow. In many uncomplicated situations, however, the only source of flow will be pressure, and flow will follow the pressure.

Concepts in Flow

"Flow" is an umbrella term that covers a lot of different meanings, as: Doppler spectral display, Doppler frequency distribution across a vessel lumen, velocity profile across a vessel lumen, and volume of blood traveling through a cardiovascular compartment. Keeping things sorted out will certainly require careful use of the words that modify "flow," as well as the physical events involved.

From Chapter 4, it is clear that the velocity across the lumen of a vessel or pipe with a steady-state flow is not uniform. If the pipe is rigid and straight, the flow profile across the lumen will be a parabola, placing the highest velocity in the center of the pipe. If the Doppler angle is constant with respect to the pipe, then examining such a flow pattern with a pulsed-Doppler device should produce a mix of frequencies that represent the velocity profile of the blood.

The ability to determine the real velocity profile by pulsed-Doppler analysis is a function of the sample volume size. The larger the sample volume, the more blurred the profile appears to be. If the sample volume is the same size as the vessel, then the ability to determine the spatial velocity profile is completely gone, but the spectrum will contain all of the Doppler shift frequencies. Under the proper conditions, then, Doppler-based analysis can estimate the distribution of Doppler shift frequencies. It can even estimate the range of speeds (velocities without a directional component). At the same time, it cannot show how the speeds are distributed in space. Whether the sample volume is large or small, the pulsed-Doppler system is blind to true velocity.

On the other hand, color flow imaging and angiodynography are introducing a new factor to blood flow analysis: an ability to see the two-dimensional flow patterns within the scanning field. This new information about spatial velocity patterns opens the door to more accurate use of normalizing concepts such as flow velocity, which does not require any additional qualifiers such as the Doppler angle and transmitting frequency.

A primary way of dealing with flow is to measure the volume of fluid traveling down a pipe per unit time. In a blood vessel, this is called volume flow; in the heart, cardiac output. Because the function of the vascular system is to deliver blood, lesions that reduce either volume flow in a vessel or cardiac output will attract attention. In the vascular system, a 50% decrease in diameter starts reducing flow through that vessel. And in the heart, one of the first indications of cardiac disease is often a decrease in cardiac output.[2] Cardiac output is also a means of looking at the functional reserve of the heart.

In a simple flow situation, the volume of fluid entering an inflexible pipe is equal to the volume that flows out of that pipe. The volume of fluid traveling down the pipe per unit time is defined by the area of the pipe and the distance the fluid moves during a fixed time period. Movement or distance over a fixed time period is really velocity. Because the spatial velocity of a fluid is not uniform over the pipe lumen, we need to use a spatial average velocity to calculate flow

$$Q = V_{avg} A \qquad (10.1)$$

where Q is the volume flow rate, V_{avg} is the spatial average velocity, and A is the pipe cross sectional area.

Under these conditions, the pressure, volume flow rate, and resistance offered by the pipe to fluid flow are related through an equation that looks a great deal like Ohm's law in electricity

$$Q = P/R \qquad (10.2)$$

where Q is the flow rate in volume (distance^3) per unit time, P is the pressure in force per unit area, and resistance (R) appears in rather complicated units of force times seconds per distance.

These equations are a two-step process to measure flow and evaluate what it means. First, measuring the average spatial velocity and the diameter (which becomes area) of a pipe provides a direct calculation of volume flow. The second equation brings together those variables that affect the volume flow, namely, the pressure driving the fluid through the pipe and the pipe's resistance to flow.

When the driving pressure and flow become pulsatile, determining volume flow requires the inclusion of both spatial and time-dependent processes. Ultimately, both spatial and time-averaged calculations are used. The spatial calculation requires knowing the contribution of all the velocity vectors to the fluid movement. For time averages, a time variable is integrated over some time interval and the result is divided by that time interval. This gives the temporal average. (For those not well versed in integral calculus, the integration of a function is equivalent to calculating the area under the curve, which in this case is a value changing over time. Dividing the resulting area by the integration time interval gives the value of the function as if it were constant over that time interval.) Figure 10-1 shows graphically how this calculation goes together.

Spatial averages come by applying the same sort of integration, but over space rather than time. Now the variable is how the velocity changes over the lumen of a vessel. The integration determines the area under the curve. Dividing by the spatial interval (the vessel diameter in this case) produces an average velocity. It is as if the velocity were constant over the lumen. Figure 10-2 depicts this calculation graphically.

Laminar flow through a vessel requires a spatial average of that flow to eventually compute the volume blood flow. In some vessels, however, the entry of flow into the vessel produces a very blunt or flat velocity flow profile. A good example of this is in the ascending aorta, for which the maximum velocity from a CW Doppler device can be used to calculate the volume flow because the velocity profile is very blunt. The details of this particular calculation appear later in the discussion.

Quantitation in Cardiology

One of the first and strikingly successful applications of Doppler quantitation was measuring cardiac output. This calculation, however, requires the correct view of the heart.

View of the Heart

Evaluating heart function centers on treating the heart as a pump. The valves in the heart must open to permit chamber filling and emptying while imposing very little resistance to the blood flowing through them. When closed, these same valves must form a fluid-tight seal, preventing retrograde flow from vessels to chambers and between chambers. In the end, the heart valves ensure a unidirectional flow of blood through the heart.

Placing a catheter in the heart's chambers permits a direct measurement of pump parameters such as cardiac output and stroke volume, pressure gradients across valves, and visualizing valve opening areas using radiopaque dyes and x-ray film. Placing dye in a downstream chamber and looking for its retrograde motion provide both an indication of regurgitation and an estimate of its severity.[3] It is precisely the ability to get at these parameters with a Doppler system that stimulated its use in the heart.

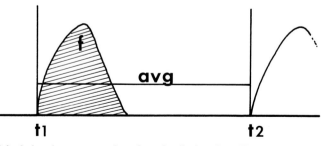

Figure 10-1   Calculating the average value of a pulsatile function. The average value is equal to the area (*shaded*) under the curve (*f*) divided by the time interval (*t1* to *t2*). The result is a value (*avg*) with the same area under it as the function (*f*).

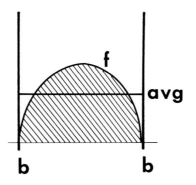

Figure 10-2 Calculating the spatial average of a velocity profile. The average value (*avg*) is equal to a value with the same area underneath as the function (*f*) over the same boundaries (*b*).

The first evaluation of the heart as a pump involves determining stroke volume and cardiac output. Furthermore, measuring the pressure gradient across a stenotic valve shows how much the valve is impeding the blood flow. Tracing how far a valve's regurgitation jet reaches into an upstream chamber not only reveals the regurgitation, but also expresses the severity of valve leakage.

Stroke Volume and Cardiac Output

The ascending or descending aorta are good sites for measuring stroke volume and cardiac output. The accelerating blood flow out of the left ventricle blunts the aortic velocity profile across the vessel.[4] This flat profile eliminates the need to make a spatial average velocity calculation. All that is needed is to follow the maximum Doppler shift frequency over the cardiac cycle.

Converting the maximum Doppler shift frequency into the maximum blood velocity uses a transposed Doppler equation

$$V = (Df\,C)/(2\,F_0 \cos \theta) \tag{10.3}$$

where V is the calculated velocity; Df is the Doppler shift frequency; F_0 is the transmit frequency; C is the ultrasound velocity of propagation; and θ is the Doppler angle. If we look at the blood flow in the ascending aorta from the suprasternal notch, the Doppler angle is close to zero. This means $\cos \theta$ is very slow changing and nearly a value of one. All the other parameters in the equation are either known or constants.

The electrocardiogram (ECG) interval between successive ECG R-waves is called the R-R interval, normally expressed in seconds. The average flow over an R-R interval, then, is

$$V_{max(avg)} = \int (V_{max}(t)\,dt)/R\text{-}R \tag{10.4}$$

where $V_{max(avg)}$ is the average maximum velocity and $V_{max}(t)$ is the time-varying, instantaneous maximum velocity. The essentials of this calculation are shown in Figure 10-3.

The stroke volume equation looks like

$$SV = A\,V_{max(avg)}\,R\text{-}R \tag{10.5}$$

where SV is the stroke volume in milliliters; A is the aortic cross sectional area; $V_{max(avg)}$ is the average maximum velocity; and R-R is the heartbeat interval in seconds. The

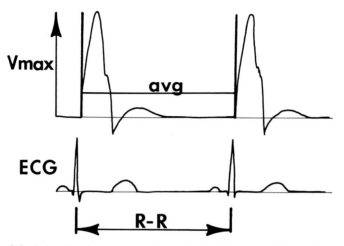

Figure 10-3   Calculating the time-average flow velocity. This calculation begins with the time course of the maximum velocity (*Vmax*). The area under the *Vmax* curve divided by the *R-R* interval (*ECG*) produces the average value (*avg*).

product of the first two terms gives the average volume flow. Multiplying by the R-R interval limits this calculation to a single heartbeat.

The basic relationship between stroke volume and cardiac output is

$$CO = (SV) (HR) \qquad (10.6)$$

where *CO* is the cardiac output in liters per minute; *SV* is the stroke volume in liters; and *HR* is the heart rate in beats per minute. The heart rate in beats per minute is related to the R-R interval by

$$HR = 60/R\text{-}R \qquad (10.7)$$

Substituting for *SV* and *HR* produces

$$CO = A\ V_{max(avg)}\ (R\text{-}R)\ (60/R\text{-}R) \qquad (10.8)$$

Unfortunately, the units for this equation are in cubic centimeters per minute. Simplifying the equation and dividing by 1,000 ml converts the equation to liters per minute. The final equation for cardiac output is

$$CO = A\ V_{max(avg)}\ (60/1000) \qquad (10.9)$$

Central to an accurate estimate of cardiac output is the measurement of the aortic area. Clearly, the aortic diameter measurement and the site of Doppler velocity measurements must be the same for these calculations to work best. In addition, errors in any diameter measurement are squared into the calculation. As a result, even small errors in diameter can have much larger effects on the calculated cardiac output. Even with these errors, coupling on-line calculations with a Doppler spectrum permits a beat-by-beat depiction of cardiac output. The real-time format is then able to show normal and abnormal changes in this physiological variable. Figure 10-4 graphs the percent error in cardiac output calculations that can result from errors in diameter measurement.

If accurate aortic diameter measurements are impossible, the clinician can still use the Doppler information expressed in units of distance. For example, the integral of the maximum velocity over the R-R interval is the stroke "distance."[5] This is hypothetically how far the blood would have traveled at its average spatial velocity during

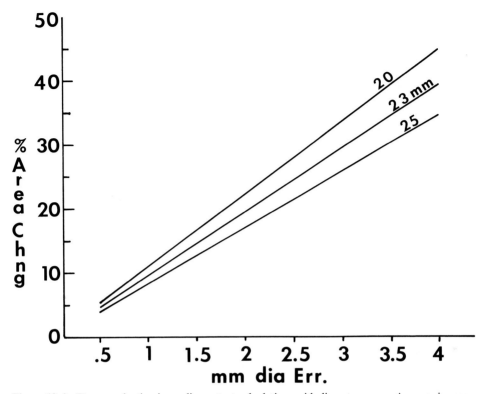

Figure 10-4   Error production in cardiac output calculations with diameter errors. An error in measuring the aortic diameter (*mm dia Err.*) produces a rapid error in the area calculation (*% Area Chng*).

the R-R interval. Of course, this concept can also include a cardiac output "distance."[6] Although these parameters are frequently used in many cardiology facilities, the terms remain unfamiliar to many and are intellectually uncomfortable to use.

The value in watching cardiac output or stroke volume on a beat-to-beat basis lies in the ability to follow the compensation of a cardiovascular system in health and disease without putting the patient at any substantive risk. The alternative is to look at the snapshots of cardiac function offered by more invasive measures of the heart, for example, indicator dilution techniques.

Valve Pressure Gradients

One way of quantifying the ability of a cardiac valve to open is to measure the pressure difference across that valve when blood flows through the opening. The traditional way to get this information is to measure the pressure on either side of the valve with a catheter. Despite the comfort of a direct measurement, it does require invading the vascular system, with some risk to the patient. A noninvasive evaluation of this parameter has real appeal and value.

Doppler processing will let us estimate this measurement after some simplifications of the Bernoulli equation and some limitations on the character of the flow. At the outset, flow through the valve must be laminar, and the flow velocities must fall below values that would make viscous forces a significant part of the flow process.[1] In general, as the stenotic valve orifice becomes smaller, the blood velocity through the valve increases. When the velocity becomes too high, however, the Doppler pressure gradient equation systematically underestimates the pressure gradient.[1] Correlation studies between direct measurements and Doppler estimates show that the latter misses the mark when the orifice diameter is less than 3.5 mm.[1]

The most successful applications of this technique are on the aortic, mitral, and tricuspid valves. The pulmonary valve is more difficult simply because it is hard to image from either the suprasternal or subcostal locations.

The calculation for pressure gradients across valves comes from the Bernoulli equation and appears as follows:

$$dP = 4 \, V_{max}^2 \tag{10.10}$$

where V_{max} is the maximum velocity of the transvalvular jet expressed in meters per second, and dP is the pressure gradient in millimeters of mercury (mmHg).

This surprisingly simple equation begins with the much larger underpinnings of the Bernoulli equation in the following manner:

$$P_1 + [(p \, v_1^2)/2] + Rv_1 = P_2 + [(p \, v_2^2)/2] + Rv_2 \tag{10.11}$$

Regrouping gives:

$$P_1 - P_2 = [p \, (v_2^2 - v_1^2)/2] + R \, (v_2 - v_1) \tag{10.12}$$

where P is the pressure on either side of the valve, p is the blood density, R is the viscosity resistance term, v_1 is the velocity entering the stenosis, and v_2 is the velocity at the outflow of the stenosis.

If v_1 is a lot smaller than v_2, then we can safely eliminate the v_1 term. The same is true of the resistance terms if the kinetic energy happens to be a great deal larger than the resistance term. The greatest pressure value occurs when the outflow velocity is at maximum, and v_2 can be rewritten as V_{max}. The equation then becomes

$$P_1 - P_2 = dP = (p/2) \, V_{max}^2 \tag{10.13}$$

where dP is the pressure difference across the stenosis. The final form of the equation emerges from some conversion factors that will permit expressing the pressure in mmHg and the maximum velocity in meters per second. It starts with the blood density, which is:

$$p = 1.06 \times 10^3 \, \text{kg/m}^3 \tag{10.14}$$

The velocity term is in meters per second (m/s). Following Eq. 10.13, density is divided by 2, which gives

$$p/2 = 0.53 \times 10^3 \, \text{kg/m3}. \tag{10.15}$$

Pressure has the units of Newtons per square meter, also expressed as kg · m/s². In addition, 1 mmHg = 133.3 N/m², thus

$$[0.53 \times 10^3 \, \text{kg} \cdot \text{m/s}^2) \, (1/\text{m}^2)]/ \, 133.3 \, \text{N/m}^2/\text{mmHg} = 3.975 \tag{10.16}$$

Therefore,

$$dP = 3.975 \, V_{max}^2$$
$$\text{or } dP = 4 \, V_{max}^2. \tag{10.17}$$

One of the major assumptions in measuring the jet velocity is that jet formation is axial to the valve geometry. With no additional information about the flow pattern, this is not a bad assumption, although nonaxial flow could greatly affect the accuracy of any gradient estimate. Color flow imaging in the heart, however, has shown that jets are frequently not axial to the valve.[7] When these variations in geometry are taken into account for calculations, the correlation between the invasive and noninvasive measurements appears to improve, with less randomness in the correlation. The basic elements of this measurement are shown in Figure 10-5.

Estimating Valve Areas

Estimating valve areas really applies only to the aortic and mitral valves. As in the pressure gradient calculation, measurements center on the maximum velocity waveform. The calculations use two different approaches; nevertheless, both estimates are based on the relationships among flow, velocity, and the area of an orifice. As shown earlier, the basic equation is:

$$Q = A \, V_{avg} \tag{10.1}$$

where Q (the volume flow rate) has the dimensions of volume per unit time; V_{avg} (spatial average fluid velocity) has the dimensions of length per unit time; and A (area) has the dimensions of length squared.

If we look at the flow over a specific period of time, such as the interval of one heartbeat, the volume of blood traveling through the valve orifice is

$$Q = A \, V_{max(avg)} \, dT \tag{10.18}$$

where Q has the dimensions of volume (length cubed), and dT is a time interval such as the R-R interval.

Aortic Valve Area Q can become the stroke volume when $V_{max(avg)}$ extends over a heart cycle or over just the ejection period within a heartbeat. The stroke volume equation is

$$SV = A \, V_{max(ejection \ avg)} \, SEP \tag{10.19}$$

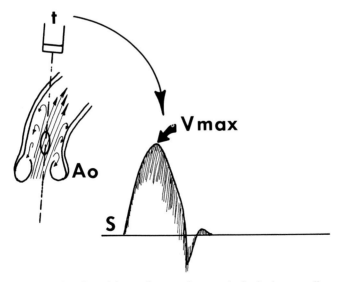

Figure 10-5   Doppler estimating of the outflow maximum velocity in the ascending aorta. *Ao* is the aorta, *t* is the transducer, *S* is the signal, and *Vmax* is the maximum velocity.

where *SEP* is the systolic ejection period, and $V_{max(ejection\ avg)}$ is averaged over the same time period. A is the aortic valve area in this case. This equation is quite useful in estimating the degree of stenosis in a diseased aortic valve.[8] Transposing the equation and solving for the area term produces

$$AVA = SV/(V_{max(avg)}\ SEP) \tag{10.20}$$

where *AVA* is the aortic valve area; *SV* is the cardiac stroke volume; $V_{max(avg)}$ is the average maximum transvalvular velocity; and *SEP* is the systolic ejection period. The central elements of these calculations are shown in Figure 10-6.

Calculating the *AVA* clearly requires a measurement of stroke volume, average maximum velocity, and systolic ejection period. The stroke volume information would most likely come from some other technique such as thermal dilution.[9] It would be difficult for the *SV* information to come from Doppler analysis because aortic valve stenosis would disrupt the flow pattern so much that the assumption of blunt flow in the ascending aorta would not be true. Conversely, if flow could be measured in the descending aorta where turbulence or disturbed flow has disappeared, then Doppler analysis can be used noninvasively to determine cardiac output and stroke volume. Cardiac output could also come from a thermal dilution measurement in the right ventricle, which would permit a calculation without left ventricle catheterization. The central elements of this calculation are shown in Figure 10-6.

Mitral Valve Area   Estimating the mitral valve area depends upon the relationship between the valve area and the rate at which the blood pressure falls in the left atrium.

A corresponding model for this situation is a closed volume that experiences increased pressure and then has a small orifice opened. The pressure in the receiving

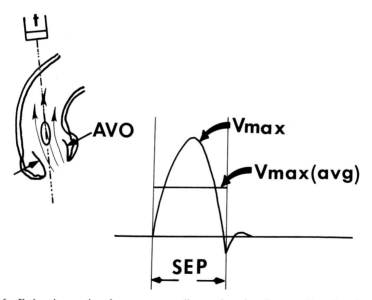

Figure 10-6   Estimating aortic valve pressure gradient and aortic valve area. Based on the Bernoulli principle, the maximum systolic velocity (*Vmax*) over the systolic ejection period (*SEP*) can be used to estimate the transvalvular pressure. The average velocity over the ejection period [*Vmax(avg)*] times the aortic root area and *SEP* gives the stroke volume. *t* is the transducer, and *AVO* is the aortic valve opening.

chamber (left ventricle) is much lower than in the source chamber (left atrium). Under these conditions, it is assumed that the pressure gradient decreases at a rate following the volume of fluid leaving the left atrium. This is a nonlinear relationship for moderate to severe stenosis, with the best calculations using the time it takes to reach half the peak pressure (hence the pressure half-times).[10]

Correlating the pressure half-time with the mitral valve area produces a nonlinear relationship that looks like a hyperbola. The general equation for a hyperbola is

$$x y = k \tag{10.21}$$

where the constant k can have any sign. A similar relationship exists for frequency and wave length, with the velocity of propagation as a constant. Using empirical relationships, the equation for estimating the effective mitral valve area (*MVA*) becomes:

$$MVA = 220/\text{pressure half-time} \tag{10.22}$$

where the pressure half-time is in milliseconds and *MVA* is in units of square centimeters.[1]

We can not measure pressure noninvasively, however. We need a relationship between the driving pressure gradient and velocity:

$$dP = 4V_{max}^2 \tag{10.23}$$
$$dP/2 = 4V_{max}^2/2$$
$$dP/2 = 4(V_{max}/\sqrt{2})^2.$$

Thus, the pressure drops by half in the time it takes for the maximum velocity to drop to 71% ($1/\sqrt{2}$). The elements of this mitral valve area measurement are illustrated in Figure 10-7.

Correlations with angiographic measurements of mitral valve area show this to be a reasonable way of estimating valve area for moderate to severe stenoses.[11] The only overt limitation is the error produced by the increasing influence of blood viscosity on the jet as a result of increasing velocity. A more subtle and difficult error arises from a jet that deviates from the central axis of the valve. Only a very careful point-by-point map of the jet pattern or color flow imaging can detect and somewhat correct this error.

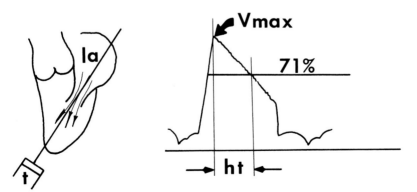

Figure 10-7   Estimating the mitral valve area from pressure half-times. As the left atrium (*la*) empties into the left ventricle, the transvalvular pressure decreases. The time to reach half-pressure (*ht*) is related to the maximum velocity (*Vmax*). The pressure drops to half in the same time as velocity decreases to 71% of maximum.

Estimating Vascular Disease

Vascular disease proceeds along four types of flow disruption: 1) flow obstruction through a narrowing of a vessel lumen; 2) vessel trauma, causing anatomical defects; 3) vasospasm; and 4) emboli that form at one location and travel to another location to obstruct flow there.

The diagnostic tools used to look at the vascular system are directed at these events. Angiography, for example, looks at the vascular compartment by delineating the lumen with radiopaque dye. Evidence for disease is a narrowed or expanded lumen. Staging the stenosis requires an estimate of the percent reduction in the lumen diameter or cross-sectional area. In addition, disruptions of the vessel intimal surface that erode into the tunica media (ulcers) may be visible in the angiogram.

Doppler analysis, on the other hand, detects and evaluates the amount of vascular disease by assessing its effects on blood flow. Narrowing a vascular lumen increases the velocity of the blood flow through the constriction, which increases the maximum Doppler shift frequencies perceived by a Doppler system. When the flow velocity increases, other flow disturbances occur that also increase the number of Doppler shift frequencies present in the echo signal, producing spectral broadening.

The central assumption, then, in the Doppler detection and evaluation of vascular disease, is that stenotic disease produces flow disturbances and as stenosis progresses, the degree of flow disturbance increases.[12] If this assumption is true, then quantitating the amount of flow disturbance can bracket the amount of stenotic disease. In most cases, this assumption holds, and studies measuring the sensitivity (the ability to detect disease in a diseased population) of a duplex Doppler scan produce values as high as 98% or so.[13] Typical values hover around 90% for the better laboratories. The cases in which this assumption does not hold true represent the false positives and false negatives yielded by Doppler and duplex studies. The false positive rate for duplex imaging, for example, is relatively high, with an 85% specificity (the ability to define normal within a population of normals).[13] Clearly, this approach cannot always distinguish an unusual normal flow pattern from one produced by disease.

Despite these limitations, Doppler analysis can detect arterial disease and categorize it generally into ranges of stenosis.[13] This is especially true of the carotid arteries, which have received a great deal of clinical attention. Other vessels are less quantifiable, and detection of disease often depends on measuring the vascular flow pulsatility.

The Carotid Arteries

Efforts to estimate the amount of disease found in the internal carotid arteries by looking at flow events in the internal (ICA) and common (CCA) carotid arteries have produced the following criteria:[14]

1. *Normal:* Normal contour CCA [(a−b)/a ratio is > 0.5)], the ICA spectrum has a window with no broadening
2. *Minimal* (1%–15% stenosis): Abnormal CCA contour [(a−b)/a ratio is < 0.5)] with a clear window for the ICA
3. *Moderate* (16%–49% stenosis): Abnormal ICA contour with broadening throughout systole, no window, and a peak frequency generally less than 4 kHz
4. *Severe* (50%–79% stenosis): Abnormal ICA contour with a systolic peak greater than 4 kHz, marked spectral broadening, increased flow velocity

5. *Severe* (80%–99% stenosis): ICA peak systolic frequency above 4 kHz, peak, and an end diastolic frequency above 4.5 kHz
6. *Occlusion:* Common carotid flow zero or reversed in diastole, no flow in internal carotid artery

In this case, a normal contour means that the first zero slope after the peak value is located more than halfway down from the maximum. This change in shape is expressed as a form of pulsatility called the (a–b)/a ratio. An abnormal CCA contour places this inflection point less than halfway down from the maximum value. In this condition, the ratio becomes greater than 0.5. These criteria and some definitions are shown in Figure 10-8.

This approach attempts to use the shape of the Doppler flow signal to look at vascular events in a more objective manner. Numerical values such as maximum frequency and the amount of spectral broadening, expressed as a percent window, can come from some computer assistance. Still, as a tool, the computer is better used for handling cumbersome calculations than as a pattern recognition system. Let's look at two of these computer algorithms that can tell us about carotid artery stenosis.

The Keagy Algorithm   In 1982, Blair A. Keagy et al.[15] introduced a quantitative approach to estimating internal carotid artery stenosis. This systematic evaluation of carotid disease relies on a combination of relative values and a quantified pattern of events over the cardiac cycle. The relative values come from comparing hydrodynamic events within a diseased internal carotid artery versus a nondiseased common carotid artery.[15] The quantified pattern comes from measuring the maximum frequency of the carotid waveforms at selected times. Using these general principles, the algorithm examines three variables (see Fig. 10-9).

The first variable is an examination of the maximum frequency present at 50%, 70%, and 90% of the cardiac cycle.[15] This places the measurements in the diastolic portion of the cardiac cycle and examines the flow rate sustained during diastole.

The second variable is a ratio of the spectral area within the internal carotid waveform to the spectral area within the common carotid artery (assumed to be disease free).[15] As a stenosis tightens, increasing both the flow velocities and amount of flow disturbance, the area covered by spectral broadening in a spectral waveform increases.

The third variable is a ratio of the peak systolic frequency at the internal carotid artery to that of the common carotid artery.[15] This is a common evaluation parameter

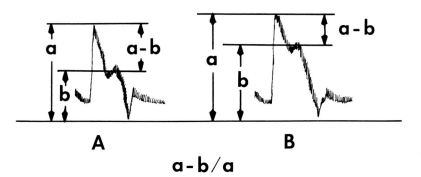

Figure 10-8   Common carotid artery contour changes with internal carotid artery disease. The *a-b/a* ratio changes in response to distal internal carotid stenosis. **A,** A normal contour has a ratio greater than 0.5. **B,** Disease decreases the ratio to less than 0.5.

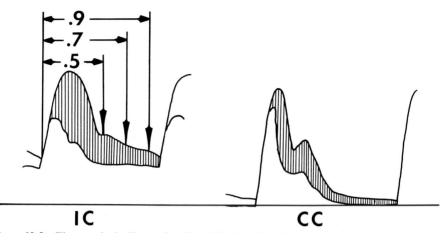

Figure 10-9   Elements in the Keagy algorithm. This algorithm depends upon the comparison of flow in a diseased internal carotid artery (*IC*) with that of a normal common carotid artery (*CC*). The first variable is maximum frequency present at 50%, 70%, and 90% of the cardiac cycle. The second variable compares the spectral area in the IC (*shaded*) to the CC (*shaded*). The third variable is a comparison of the peak systolic frequency in the IC and the CC.

and seems to be a good primary indicator of the elevated velocities associated with vessel stenosis, either in absolute values as in the earlier stenosis criteria, or as the relational value used here.

Values derived from the first two variables are then combined into an equation that produces a "predictive value" correlating with the presence and severity of disease.[15] These two sets of values are called test A and B. Test A is the frequency area ratio, and test B is the sum of the maximum frequencies at the three points in diastole. The values in test B are in kilohertz units but are expressed as centimeters distance on the hard copy of a spectrum. The equation is

$$V = 0.2232 \ln A + 0.1752 \ln B \qquad (10.24)$$

where V is the predictive value and ln is the natural logarithm (the base e). If V is less than 0.606, the vessel is estimated to have a less than 50% diameter reduction. This range also includes normal vessels. If V is equal to or greater than 0.606, the vessel is estimated to have a 50% to 90% diameter reduction. In use, the algorithm appears to provide a good separation of stenoses of 40% or less from those of 60% or more.[15]

Roederer-Strandness Algorithm   The Roederer-Strandness (RS) algorithm is a form of computer pattern recognition.[13] Separation of the spectral parts in this algorithm is more detailed than the Keagy approach. In addition, this algorithm requires an accumulation of data over several heartbeats for the analysis to work.

The user first collects spectral waveforms from 20 heartbeats. They are averaged to produce an ensemble spectrum, showing the form and frequency content over time and the frequency component amplitudes. The analysis then determines the *mode* of the ensemble, which is the frequency with the largest amplitude at each sampling period. Using the amplitude information, the analysis then draws contour lines that follow the frequency components above and below the mode with amplitudes -3 dB and -9 dB below maximum, as shown in Figure 10-10.

If the computer judges the pattern to be abnormal, the first decision is whether or

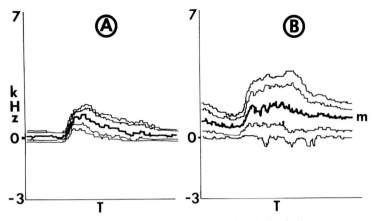

Figure 10-10 Roederer-Strandness computer-based spectral analysis. **A,** A computer-generated frequency analysis from an ensemble of spectra low on a normal common carotid artery. **B,** A similar ensemble frequency analysis from the proximal portion of an internal carotid artery with severe disease. The Y-axis is frequency in kHz. The dark center line (*m*) is the mode frequency. The next outer pair of lines are the frequencies − 3 dB below the mode, and the next pair are − 9 dB below the mode. (Courtesy of Department of Surgery, University of Washington School of Medicine, Seattle, Washington.)

not the results suggest stenosis above or below 50%. If the indication is a stenosis less than 50%, then the analysis determines if the value is greater or less than 20%. The decision steps in the algorithm use some 15 parameters within the contour waveforms to arrive at specific classifications.[13] The overall performance of this analytical technique has been very good, with the authors reporting a 97% sensitivity (ability to detect disease) and a 93% specificity (ability to show normals).[13]

RS versus Keagy Algorithms   A comparison between these two approaches to evaluating carotid artery disease will show some of the strengths and weaknesses of these two techniques.

The first RS algorithm divides the full range of occlusive disease into six stages, including normal and occluded. Although its accuracy in determining the presence or absence of disease (sensitivity) may be high, the actual staging of disease into the various levels can be much less precise. Deriving some understanding about the degree of stenosis requires a detailed look at the spectral recordings.

In contrast, the Keagy algorithm sets out to divide the full range of carotid artery disease into either hemodynamically significant or insignificant, i.e., above or below 50% (diameter) stenosis. In fact, the best separation occurs with stenoses less than 40% and greater than 60%. In general, this approach requires less human analysis and offers more computer-based assistance in the evaluation.

These two approaches are in fact asking different questions about the same occlusive carotid artery disease. Still, they both examine the dynamics of the blood flow to determine how much disease may be present. Because the Keagy algorithm has a more mathematical approach, its binary division of disease classes may show the real blurring that normally occurs when we try to stage carotid artery disease. The blurring comes from the superposition of an adaptive vascular system onto the progressively obstructive disease, and all the errors inherent in the measurement process.

Examining Other Arteries

Assessing the condition of a distal vascular bed can require a very detailed analysis. It could require examining individual branches within a vascular bed, which is a rather sizable problem to solve. Unfortunately, the vascular system is not simple enough for such a detailed approach. A more generalized way of looking at these vascular beds is to examine the hydraulic response of the bed to an approaching pulse wave. By measuring how the pulse wave changes, we can get some idea of the downstream conditions. This is the logic behind the notion of measuring pulsatility.

Four different pulsatility calculations are currently used for vascular evaluations: 1) the peak-to-peak pulsatility index; 2) Pourcelot's ratio; 3) the mean pulsatility index; and 4) the (a − b)/a ratio. And beneath the umbrella words "pulsatility index" are a few variations on this central theme. The central idea behind the various indices is that an index will cancel out errors in estimation caused by the Doppler angle, machine gain settings, and patient conditions such as hypo- or hypertension. Ideally, the ratio or index should show only variations in the vascular state.

The Pulsatility Index The first version of this parameter was the Fourier pulsatility index. The calculation of this parameter is based on the Fourier components of the *maximum* blood flow velocity waveform.[16] The Fourier series of this waveform can be described as

$$V(t) = V_0/2 + \sum_{n=1}^{\infty} [V_n \cos(nwt\text{-}A_n)] \tag{10.25}$$

where $V(t)$ is the time function of the maximum velocity, V_0 is the mean forward velocity of the wave form, n is the harmonic number from 1 to infinity, V_n is the nth harmonic of the velocity waveform, w is the heart rate expressed as an angular frequency (radians per second), and A_n is the phase angle of the nth harmonic.

The Fourier pulsatility index (PI_F) is

$$PI_F = \sum_{n=1}^{\infty} [V_n^2 / V_0^2] \tag{10.26}$$

where the values of V_n and V_0 are squared.[16] Energy is proportional to the square of velocity, so these squared terms take the form of energy. The numerator is the maximum oscillatory energy of the wave and the denominator is the energy of the mean forward flow.

Attempts to use this index have shown that it estimates the severity of occlusive arterial disease that had been detected using arteriograms, pressure measurements at the ankle, and blood flow measurements into a limb.[16] Because this calculation is not automated in any sonographs, it remains difficult and time consuming and not widely used for that reason.

Peak-to-Peak Pulsatility Index The peak-to-peak pulsatility index uses the total excursion of the waveform and its mean value to look at the time course of the pulse.[17] The calculation of this index has the form

$$PI_{pp} = \text{peak-to-peak velocity/mean velocity.} \tag{10.27}$$

This parameter is generally independent of the Doppler angle over a rather wide range of angles. The calculation is usually carried out using the maximum velocity or frequency waveform. The graphic character of the measurement is shown in Figure 10-11.

Attempts to link the Fourier pulsatility index with the peak-to-peak version show a close kinship.[16] If the form of a maximum velocity profile is a mean forward flow, V_0, with a sinusoidal waveform superimposed, then the following relationship holds:

$$PI_{pp} = 2 \, (PI_F)^{0.5} \tag{10.28}$$

Actually making measurements and determining the relationship between PI_{pp} and PI_F yields a regression equation:[16]

$$PI_{pp} = 1.9 \, (PI_F)^{0.57} \tag{10.29}$$

Thus, the peak-to-peak index should have a sensitivity similar to that shown by the Fourier version.

Because the calculation of the PI_{pp} is straightforward, it is frequently found on dedicated vascular sonographs. It can also be used to calculate a damping factor, based on the observation that the PI_{pp} normally increases as we look at increasingly distal vessels.[18] In contrast, the presence of occlusive disease proximal to the measurement site *decreases* the index. This is a consequence of the distal vasculature dilating to compensate for the proximal stenosis. Thus, calculating a progressive damping factor may be able to detect a peripheral vascular obstruction proximal to the measurement site. This calculation, however, tends to increase with the severity of the occlusion, so an inverse damping factor is often used to show a decreasing index with increasing disease.

PI_{pp} is a parameter that responds best to changes in a high-resistance vascular bed. The range of values for PI_{pp} is 0.0 to 15, with the higher values around 12. As the vascular bed decreases resistance, the diastolic flow increases, decreasing the peak-to-peak value, resulting in a slow changing mean value.

Pourcelot's Ratio   An alternate way of looking at vascular pulsatility is to examine the differences between the systolic and diastolic periods of the pulse. Pourcelot's ratio is such an index of pulsatility, calculated as follows:[17]

$$PR = (S - D) / S \tag{10.30}$$

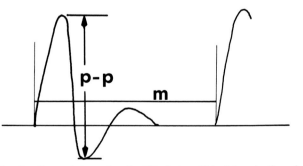

Figure 10-11   Estimating the peak-to-peak pulsatility index. This determination of pulsatility works best in high-resistance vascular beds. The index results from measuring the peak-to-peak value (*p-p*) and dividing it by the mean value (*m*) over the cardiac cycle. Values do not exceed 12 under typical biological conditions.

where S is the peak systolic velocity (or frequency) and D is the minimum or end diastolic velocity (or frequency). The elements of this ratio are shown in Figure 10-12.

This is a simple and direct way of looking at vascular events and tends to be independent of the Doppler angle. This independence may not hold when the angle is close to 90°, however, and the diastolic frequencies become too low for display. Because the calculation is easy and direct, this ratio is often found in the software calculation packages in vascular sonographs.

In general, Pourcelot's ratio is suitable for low-resistance vascular beds with flow in diastole. If the end-diastolic value (D) goes to zero, the ratio converges to one, and further changes in vascular resistance do not change the ratio. Values range, then, from 0.0 to 1.0.

The Mean Pulsatility Index   A pulsatility index with growing applications for renal transplants is the mean pulsatility index. This parameter uses selective parts of PI_{pp} and PR to extend its useful range of application. The index takes the form

$$PI_{mean} = (S - D)/\text{mean} \tag{10.31}$$

where PI_{mean} is the mean pulsatility index, S is the peak systolic velocity (or frequency), D is the end-diastolic velocity (or frequency), and "mean" is the mean value over the cardiac cycle. Clearly, the numerator of this equation came from Pourcelot's ratio, and the denominator came from the PI_{pp} equation.

This parameter handles a much wider range of resistance changes than either PI_{pp} or PR. Because of the large changes in vascular resistance that can occur in renal transplants, this is an often used ratio.

The (a − b)/a Ratio   A ratio often used to determine whether a common carotid artery waveform is near normal or not is the (a − b)/a ratio.[13] This calculation really tests for the presence and timing of the dichrotic inflection of the carotid artery waveform. It is used in the RS algorithm as one of the tests for a normal carotid waveform.[13] The ratio (R) is calculated as:

$$R = (a - b) / a \tag{10.32}$$

where a is the peak systolic frequency, and b is the peak frequency at the inflection of the carotid waveform. This is mathematically the location of the first zero slope, that is,

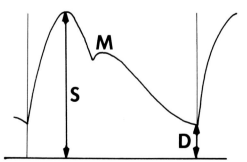

Figure 10-12   Estimating Pourcelot's ratio. This measure of pulsatility seems to work best in low-resistance vascular beds that have diastolic flow. The ratio becomes zero when the peak systolic (S) and end diastolic (D) frequencies or velocities are equal. The ratio is 1 when the diastolic value becomes zero.

where the waveform turns around near the end of systole. Ratios above 0.5 are considered normal, below 0.5 are abnormal, ranging from mild to severe disease. The graphic elements of this calculation are shown in Figure 10-8.

Laplace Transforms

A particularly successful way of handling difficult differential equations is to transform them into a form that permits an easy, algebraic solution. One such transformation is called the Laplace transform, which changes a time-domain equation (an equation with units of time) into a frequency-domain equation (an equation with units of frequency) with a simple algebraic form.[19] This turns out to be a very different approach as well to the analysis problems integral to evaluating peripheral vascular disease.

The vascular application of this transformation begins with collecting the velocity time course of blood flow through a peripheral vessel using a Doppler sonograph.[20] This waveform is then digitized and passed through a FFT circuit to obtain the Fourier frequency components of the velocity waveform. The frequency components then pass through a second transformation, the Laplace transformation. This transformation is found empirically by curve fitting a transform of the form[20]

$$1/(S^3 + AS^2 + BS + C) \tag{10.33}$$

where S in Equation 10.33 is the complex angular frequency jw and j is the square root of -1. (A complex number is a number composed of real and mathematically imaginary parts. The square root of -1 is undefined and therefore imaginary.) The Laplace transform changes the complicated differential equation used to describe flow in the vascular system into a simpler algebraic expression for easy solution. In this case, A, B, and C are coefficients that are experimentally determined for the best curve fit.

Through some rigorous clinical correlations, the solutions to such an equation relate back to physical parameters in the vessels. They include qualities such as arterial stiffness, peripheral impedance, and lumen size.[20] And these are certainly parameters that can represent the physical state of a peripheral vessel and vascular bed. Clinical recordings from vessels, such as the posterior tibial artery in patients with total occlusion of the superficial femoral artery, correctly predict collateralization.[20] In addition, this technique can distinguish disease that is either proximal or both proximal and distal to the Doppler sampling site.[20]

Like many of the other calculations and analyses of pulsatility, this technique requires substantial computer support. In addition, the connection between the analytical results and clinical conclusions is based on complex, mathematical relationships. Despite the quality of the Laplace transform, widespread clinical use will depend upon its incorporation and automation in future Doppler sonographs.

Calculations and Errors

Despite our natural obsession with quantitating the clinical results of Doppler analysis, quantitation is not without some logic and calculation traps. Within any calculation are assumptions about the nature of the flow pattern as well as errors that propagate through nonlinear equations. And false conclusions about the accuracy of an approach can result from using measurements that affect the parameter being measured. At the center of most calculations is an assumption about the character of flow.

Flow Assumptions

Many calculations make assumptions about the pattern of flow within a vascular compartment. A cardiac output calculation using flow in the ascending aorta, for example, assumes a blunt velocity pattern. Volume flow measurements in smaller vessels, on the other hand, assume a laminar flow pattern with the maximum velocity moving down the center of the vessel. Greater scrutiny of the range of normal flow events clearly suggest patterns that are disturbed and complex in the absence of disease.

In vascular disease, it is often assumed that the stenotic lesion forms a jet that follows the axial geometry of the vessel. In fact, atherosclerotic lesions seldom arise with axial symmetry, and the jets caused by these lesions will often be directed away from the central axis. Assuming an axial geometry that is not real is an obvious partial explanation for the scatter in Doppler data we see. This scatter shows up nicely when comparing a Doppler estimate of stenosis with estimates from angiography or visual inspections at surgery.

One of the first clues to nonaxial flow is upstream and downstream measurements of the same vessel location that are markedly different. The source of this error is shown in Figure 10-13. It was this sort of hidden Doppler angle error that may have generated the general belief that upstream measurements produce higher frequencies than downstream measurements.

Vessels are not the only place we assume axial symmetry for stenotic disease. Estimating a pressure gradient or a valve area in echocardiography requires an accurate estimate of the maximum velocity, which depends again on knowing the Doppler angle. Staging regurgitation is another example where mapping the penetration of a regurgitant jet into a cardiac chamber depends on the angle of the jet with respect to the valve central axis. One of the benefits of the more current use of color flow imaging is the three-dimensional determination of a stenotic jet's position in space. Knowing the true direction of jets in vessels and the heart improves the accuracy of estimating the amount of disease.

Computing Velocities

Doppler analysis began with Doppler sounds, which then extended into spectral analysis. Common to both these expressions of blood movement is the Doppler-shift frequency. From the Doppler equation, we know that these frequencies change not only with the changing Doppler angle, but also with the transmit frequency. Thus, expressing limits of normal blood flow as a Doppler-shift frequency must include the transmit frequency and the Doppler angle. Compounding this problem further is the wide range of Doppler systems with an equally wide range of transmit frequencies. The most obvious solution is to translate Doppler-shift frequencies into blood velocities.

The importance of determining the Doppler angle depends upon the level of accuracy expected in any calculation. If the angle is close to $0°$, then surprisingly large variations in the angle produce very small errors. For example, the cosine of $5°$ is 0.996, which suggests that an angular error of plus or minus $5°$ produces a velocity error in the order of plus or minus 1.5%. In contrast, at an angle of $60°$, a variation in $5°$ can produce an error in the order of plus or minus 15%. Table 10-1 shows the percentage of error introduced by a one degree angle error for various Doppler angles. The error production is small near $0°$, and very large near $80°$ and above.

If the jet direction is unknown within a heart or vascular compartment, this error

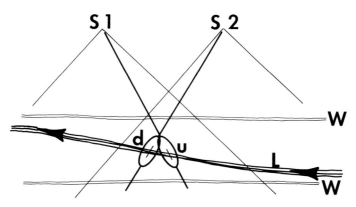

Figure 10-13 Doppler angle errors in velocity estimates. Assuming flow to be parallel to the vessel wall can generate errors if the flow is not parallel. These deviations are evident in different upstream (*u*) and downstream (*d*) Doppler frequencies as the streamline (*L*) moves from one vessel wall (*W*) to the other. *S1* and *S2* are different sector scanning fields.

can begin to grow to significant levels. Even if the error is suspected, it is almost undetectable with conventional duplex devices. One way of improving a velocity estimate is to decrease the size of the sample volume and map out the flow complexity. This solution is better on paper than in reality, however, because mapping a complicated flow pattern with a duplex system can be frustratingly slow. In a busy practice, this can mean significant loss of revenue, not to mention operator boredom. But if the mapping is automatic, as in the case of color flow imaging and angiodynography,[21] then looking at the flow pattern in long axis and in transverse can make velocity calculations much more accurate and useful.

Inability to determine the flow direction is only one way to come up with a poor estimate of velocity. Using velocity to calculate the pressure gradient of a stenotic valve depends upon the relationship between the viscosity of the blood and the velocity it reaches when jetting through a stenotic valve.[1] If the velocity is low enough, we can

Table 10-1.   Error Rates for Velocity Calculations for Various Doppler Angles

Angle (degrees)	Percent error/degree
0	0.015
20	0.650
45	1.8
50	2.1
55	2.5
60	3.0
65	3.8
70	4.8
75	6.5
80	9.9
85	20.0
88	50.0
89	100.0

ignore the contributions of blood viscosity to the total energy consideration of the blood passing through a tight opening. When a stenosis is too small, however, increasing amounts of the energy go into overcoming the viscosity effects. The result is a consistent underestimate of the pressure gradient.[1]

Another significant, yet subtle, effect on the calculation of maximum velocities is simply the gray-scale assignments of a spectral display. If the amplitude of the maximum Doppler shift frequency is too small, it may not appear on the spectral display. Because the analyst does not know the frequency is missing, a cursor readout will simply use a lower value.

Often, a noisy spectrum will make a determination of maximum frequencies quite difficult. Trying to improve a spectral display by removing noise and low amplitude signals with a reject can also lead to an underestimate of maximum Doppler frequencies and blood velocities.

Problems in Measuring Cardiac Output

Measuring cardiac output or stroke volume using Doppler in the ascending or descending aorta rests on a central assumption that flow in the aorta is blunt. Measuring the maximum velocity of the aorta and how it changes over the cardiac cycle would be very difficult if this flow were not blunt. Fortunately, for most situations where the aortic valve is healthy, the combination of acceleration and entry effects blunt the velocity profile.

This is not the case, however, if the aortic valve is to any degree stenotic or if the valve architecture distorts the formation of the pulse wave front. When this distortion occurs, an estimated maximum velocity may not represent the spatial velocity profile across the orifice. As a result, cardiac output can appear to vary greatly. A good rule to follow here is that any signs of a flow disturbance should cast doubt on any Doppler-dependent flow measurements.

On occasion, an echocardiographer will estimate cardiac output using a CW Doppler with no information about where it happens to be sampling the aortic flow. These systems often require a second measurement of the aortic diameter to calculate the aortic volume flow. An accurate estimate requires making the diameter measurement at the same location as the maximum velocity. As it turns out, the highest velocity is not typically at the aortic root, but 1 to 2 cm above the Sinus of Valsalva. As the aorta ascends from the aortic root, the vessel narrows, and the highest velocity appears in this narrower segment. Using the highest velocity and the aortic root to represent vessel dimensions will systematically overestimate cardiac output and stroke volume.

As it turns out, the display used to measure the aortic diameter also contributes to the accuracy of the calculation. The A-mode display is the most accurate means of measuring range (the diameter in this case) with ultrasound. Unfortunately, this display is often thought to be "ancient" and absent from most of the newer sonographs. A good second choice is an M-mode, or a B-mode image if that is the only choice. The poorest is the B-mode image because of the blending of gray-scale signals at the aortic interfaces. And because these measurements are squared into an area calculation, a linear error of one or two millimeters can introduce a significant error in the output measurements. Figure 10-14 shows how these errors can grow.

Measurements using a CW Doppler without the aid of a B-mode image have an additional problem: getting into the right vessel. In some individuals, the innominate artery can be central enough to be mistaken for the ascending aorta. Because the ve-

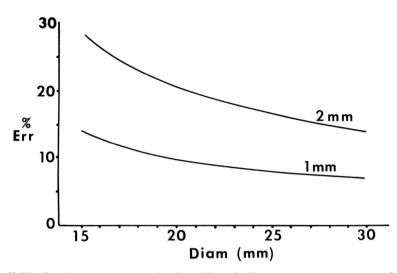

Figure 10-14 Cardiac output error production with aortic diameter measurement errors. One- and two-millimeter errors in estimating the aortic diameter introduce an error in the cardiac output calculations. As the aortic diameter becomes smaller, the percentage error (*% Err*) increases.

locities in this artery are higher than in the aorta, the calculation will overestimate cardiac output significantly. Fortunately, these two vessels have very different flow patterns, and these differences are easy to discern in the Doppler sounds and any spectral display.

Mixing Measurements

Doppler measurements of cardiac output require user skill in using the device as well as scanning the patient. Building confidence in a newly acquired Doppler technology often requires building a correlation between an invasive technique and the Doppler calculation. Thermal dilution is probably the most common of these invasive measurements.

Early attempts to correlate thermal dilution and Doppler cardiac output measurements proved to be nearly impossible. The Doppler measurements seemed to scatter more than expected. The problem was the sequence of measurements. A thermal dilution measurement introduces a cold saline indicator into the heart. The changes in blood temperature inside the ventricle indicate the washout of the indicator, which is heat (or really the lack of heat). Of course, changing the temperature of the blood also changes the temperature of the heart and its biochemistry. The result can be a decreased heart function, and this reduction showed up in the following measurements with Doppler. Reversing the sequence, on the other hand, brought the correlation much closer, and the potential for Doppler as a clinical tool became better realized.

References

1. Hatle, L, and Angelsen, B. *Doppler Ultrasound in Cardiology.* Philadelphia: Lea & Febiger, 1982, pp 24, 77, 81, 83, 185–193.
2. Sokolow, M. Heart and great vessels. *In* Krupp, MA and Chatton, MJ (eds): *Current Medical Diagnosis and Treatment,* Los Altos, CA: Lange Medical, 1983, pp 164–257.

3. Abbasi, AS, Allen, MW, DeCristofaro, D, et al. Detection and estimation of the degree of mitral regurgitation by range-gated pulsed Doppler echocardiography. *Circulation* 61: 143–147, 1980.
4. Bergel, DH. Blood flow dynamics. *In* Perronneau, P and Diebold, B (eds): *Cardiovascular Applications of Doppler Echography.* Publication 111. Paris: Institut National de la Santé et de la Recherche Medicale publication, 1982, pp 65–80.
5. Haites, NE, McLennan, FM, Mowat, DH, et al. Assessment of cardiac output by the Doppler ultrasound technique alone. *Br Heart J* 53:123–129, 1985.
6. Haites, NE, McLennan, FM, Mowat, DH, et al. How far is the cardiac output? *Lancet* 2:1025–1027, 1984.
7. Hatle, L. Noninvasive assessment and differentiation of left ventricular outflow obstruction with Doppler ultrasound. *Circulation* 64:381–387, 1981.
8. Goldberg, SJ, Sahn, DJ, Allen, HD, et al. Evaluation of pulmonary and systemic blood flow by 2-dimensional Doppler echocardiography using fast fourier transform spectral analysis. *Am J Cardiol* 50:1394–1400, 1982.
9. Libanoff, AJ, and Rodbard, S. Evaluation of the severity of mitral stenosis and regurgitation. *Circulation* 33:218–226, 1966.
10. Holen, J, Asslid, R, Landmark, K, et al. Determination of effective orifice area in mitral stenosis from non-invasive ultrasound Doppler data and mitral flow rates. *Acta Medica Scand* 201:83–88, 1977.
11. Stamm, RB, Martin, RP. Quantification of pressure gradients across stenotic valves by Doppler ultrasound. *J Am Col Card* 2:707–718, 1983.
12. Evans, TC Jr, and Taenzer, JC. Ultrasound imaging of atherosclerosis in carotid arteries. *Appl Radiol* 106–115, 1979.
13. Roederer, GO, Langlois, Y, and Strandness, DE Jr. Comprehensive noninvasive evaluation of extracranial cerebrovascular disease. *In* Hershey, FB, Barnes, RW, and Sumner, D (eds): *Noninvasive Diagnosis of Vascular Disease.* Pasadena, California: Appleton Davies, 1984, pp 177–216.
14. Langlois, Y, Roederer, GO, Chan, A, et al. Evaluating carotid artery disease, the concordance between pulsed Doppler/spectrum analysis and angiography. *Ultrasound Med Biol* 9:51–63, 1983.
15. Keagy, BA, Pharr, WF, Thomas, D, et al. A quantitative method for the evaluation of spectral analysis patterns in carotid artery stenosis. *Ultrasound Med Biol* 8:625–630, 1982.
16. Johnston, KW, Maruzzo, BC, Kassam, M, et al. Methods for obtaining, processing and quantifying Doppler blood velocity waveforms. *In* Nicolaides, AN and Yoa, JST (eds): *Investigation of Vascular Disorders.* New York: Churchill Livingston, 1981, pp 532–558.
17. Thompson, RS, Trudinger, BJ, and Cook, CM. A comparison of Doppler ultrasound waveform indices in the umbilical artery—I. Indices derived from the maximum velocity waveform. *Ultrasound Med Biol* 12:835–844, 1986.
18. Baker, AR, Evans, DH, Prytherch, DR, et al. Some failings of pulsatility index and damping factor. *Ultrasound Med Biol* 12: 875–881, 1986.
19. Kreyszig, E. *Advanced Engineering Mathematics.* New York: John Wiley, 1962, pp 205–211.
20. Atkinson, P, and Woodcock, JP. *Doppler Ultrasound and Its Use in Clinical Measurement.* New York: Academic Press, 1982, pp 189–192.
21. Powis, RL. Angiodynography: A new real-time look at the vascular system. *Appl Radiol* 15:55–59, 1986.

Index

Page numbers followed by t or f indicate tables or figures.

(a—b)/a ratio, 167f, 170, 172–173
Absorption, of beam energy, 22
Acoustical coupling, 32
  importance of, 2
Acoustical shadowing, 31–32
Acoustic impedance, mathematical definition
  of, 18
Acoustic interfaces
  definition of, 18
  reflections at, 18–22
  reflectivity of, 22–23
  relative reflectivity in decibels below per-
    fect reflector, 22–23
  strongly reflective, 22
  weakly reflective, 22
Acoustic reflectivity, 15
ADC. *See* Analog-to-digital conversion
Air, reflectivity in decibels below perfect reflector, 23t
Aliasing, 107
  definition of, 104
  high-frequency, 71, 96, 104, 105f,
    125–127, 126f
  and sampling, 125
  high PRF reduction of, 128f, 128–129
  single-line, 127, 127f
  solutions for, 127–130
  spectral signal, unwrapping, 129, 129f
A-mode imaging, of aortic diameter, 176
Analog-to-digital conversion, for FFT,
  102–103
Angiodynography, 72, 118, 123–125, 141
  of flow patterns, 150, 157, 175
Angiography, 166
Angle of insonation, 2. *See also* Doppler
  angle

in interpretation of carotid duplex
  imaging, 5
standardization to velocity criteria, 5
Annular transducer array, 90, 91f
  focusing, 151–152, 152f
Aorta
  ascending, outflow maximum velocity in,
    Doppler estimation of, 163f
  blunt velocity profile in, 141, 158
    assumptions about, 176
  diameter of, measurement errors, and car-
    diac output error production, 176, 177f
  as site for measurement of cardiac output or
    stroke volume, 159
  volume flow calculation for, 158
Aortic area, measurement of, 160–161
Aortic jet(s), non-axial, geometry of, 149,
  150f
Aortic valve
  area, estimation of, 163–164, 164f
  pressure gradient across, 162
    estimation of, 164f
  regurgitation, flow events in, 143
  stenosis, 4
Artifacts, 4–5, 7. *See also* Range ambiguity
  artifact
  from tissue-ultrasound interaction, 30–33
Atherosclerotic cervical cerebrovascular disease, ultrasound of, 7
Atherosclerotic plaque, and Doppler flow detection, 5, 174
Atrial filling, 59
Attenuation, 22. *See also* Tissue attenuation
  and penetration, 25–29
Audio output, 133
  loudness, 2–3

Autocorrelator circuit, 93–94, 95f
AVA. See Aortic valve, area
Average maximum velocity, in stroke volume
    determination, 159

Ballow, Buys, 63–64
Bandwidth, 76
Baroreceptors, 46
Baseline control, 126–127
Bats, echo-signal processing, 11–12
    capabilities and parameters of, 12, 12t
    frequencies, 12, 12t
    object size resolution, 12, 12t
Beam energy, loss of, 22
Beam focusing, in duplex system, 117, 117f
Beam steering, in duplex system, 117, 117f
Bernoulli equation, 51–53, 52f, 55, 156
    application of, 53–54
    in calculation of pressure gradient across
        valves, 162
    and energy loss through flow resistance, 53
    inertial terms in, 53
    modified, 4, 53–54
Bernoulli principle, 25
Blood
    critical Reynolds number for, 58
    effective scattering unit in, 25
    fluid behavior of, 57–58
        in heart, 59–60
        in larger vessels, 58–59
        and quantitation, 156
        at stenosis, 58, 59f, 138f, 138–139
    movement of, 135–137
    physical characteristics of, 56–60
        summary of, 60
    pressure and pulse propagation in, 39–40
    reflectivity
        in decibels below perfect reflector, 23t
        and hematocrit, 23, 24f
    ultrasound propagation velocity and at-
        tenuation rates for, 19t
    ultrasound scattering from, 56
    viscosity, effect on flow patterns, 165,
        175–176
Blood-bone interface, reflection from, 27f
Blood-brain interface, reflection from, 27f
Blood flow
    energy gradient of, 54–55, 156
    evaluation of, with color Doppler ultra-
        sound, 6
    laminar, 137, 138f
    Newtonian, 57–58
    non-Newtonian, 57
    normal, sources of spectral broadening in,
        148f–149f
    within separation bubble, 140
    sequence of events in, 135–136
    unstable, 58

velocity
    as substitute for measured Doppler shift
        frequency, 72–74
    through constriction, 166
velocity gradient, 137
velocity profile of, 156. *See also* Blunt ve-
        locity profile;
    Parabolic velocity profile
    with vessel narrowing, 138–139
Blood pressure
    systolic, measurement of, 1–2
    and vascular narrowing, 46
Blunt flow, 141
Blunt velocity profile, 49, 49f
    in aorta, 158
    of blood, 137–138, 138f
B-mode imaging, 4–5
    of aortic diameter, 176
Bone
    reflectivity in decibels below perfect reflec-
        tor, 23t
    ultrasound propagation velocity and at-
        tenuation rates for, 19t
Boundary layer, 48, 49f
    in blood flow, 137, 138f
    with unstable flow, 50
Brain, reflectivity in decibels below perfect
        reflector, 23t
Brightness, of color, 120
Bruit, 139

c. See Propagation velocity
C. See Propagation velocity
Cardiac cycle
    flow pattern in, 135–137
    vascular flow events over, 54, 55f
Cardiac output, determination of, 4, 157–161
    correlation of Doppler-derived estimates
        with invasive techniques, 177
    errors in, resulting from diameter measure-
        ment errors, 160, 161f
    problems in, 176–177
Cardiac output distance, 161
Cardiogenic shock, with vasospasm, Doppler
        sound patterns with, 3
Cardiology, quantitation in, 158–173
Cardiovascular system, as extended organ, 11
Carotid arteries. *See also* Common carotid
        artery
    anatomical variations of, 4–5
    blood flow in, 58
    disease in
        estimation of, 166–169
        grading of, 166–167
    duplex imaging, 7
        angle of insonation in, 5
        artifacts in, 4–5

nonaxial flow through, angiodynography
of, 72
occlusive disease of, 4
stenosis, computer algorithms for estimating, 167–169
Carotid bulb
flow separations in, 50–51, 51f
waveforms in, 140
Carrying material, 17
Centipoise, 43
Closing velocity, 66–68
formation of, 68f
rules governing, 67f
CO. See Cardiac output
Color Doppler ultrasound, 5–6
artifacts, 6
of atherosclerotic cervical cerebrovascular
disease, 7
errors in interpretation, 6
of extraluminal flow, 6
of pseudoaneurysms, 6
Color flow imaging, 72, 118, 122–123, 133
of flow patterns, 150–151, 157, 163, 165,
174–175
synchronous
internal organization for, 119, 120f
sampling for, 119f
using sector scanning field in, 122, 123f
Color imaging, benefits of, 121–122
Color parameters, 120–121
Color saturation, 121
Common carotid artery
contour changes with internal carotid artery disease, 167f
normal, raw Doppler signals from, 147f
Complex numbers
definition of, 104
and fast Fourier transform, 104–107
in frequency analysis, 106f, 128
Compression, in fluids, 47f
Connective tissue, ultrasound propagation velocity and attenuation rates for, 19t
Conservation of mass, 41, 45, 55, 156
Continuous wave Doppler duplex system, 90,
91f, 113f, 113–114
limitations of, 114, 115f
Continuous wave Doppler system, 75–76
amplifier, 77, 77f
combination with conventional imaging
transducers, 90, 91f
comparator, 77, 77f
limitations of, 82
organization of, 76–78, 77f
receiver, 77f
sampling fields for, 83f
signal processing in, 76–78
signal separation problem in, 94–95
spatial discrimination of, improving,
89–90

transducer pair, focused, 89–90
transducers, 89–90
operating frequency, 89–90
transmitter, 77f
Cosine Θ, 68
calculation of, 71
changes in, 71t
Coupling gel, 32
Critical velocity equation, 44
CW. *See* Continuous wave Doppler system

DAC. *See* Digital-to-analog conversion
Decibel, 33
Deep venous thrombosis, 7
Df. See Doppler shift frequency
Diagnostic imaging, color, 121–122
Diagnostic ultrasound
capabilities and parameters of, 12, 12t
frequencies, 12, 12t
object size resolution, 12, 12t
Digital-to-analog conversion, for FFT, 103
Doppler, Christian Johann, 11, 63
Doppler analysis, quantitative, 155. *See also*
Quantitation
Doppler angle, 71, 130. *See also* Cosine Θ
errors, 151
in velocity estimates, 175f, 175t
and flow velocity, 72–74
importance of, in velocity estimation, 174
real, determination of, 72
and spectral content of flow signal,
150–151
Doppler detector, 86
Doppler displays, 133. *See also* Spectral
display(s)
Doppler effect
with changing transmitting frequency,
68–69, 69f
first, 65f, 65–66
first and second, combination of, 69–70
general principle of, 10–11
initial conditions for, 64–65
in light, 63–64
in nature, 11–12
second, 65–69, 67f
in sound, 64
Doppler equation, 10
derived from phase changes associated
with moving target in echo-ranging
system, 96–97
origins of, 63–64
as tool, 63–74
use of, 70–71
Doppler operating modes, 75
Doppler physics, 9
Doppler shift frequency, 10–11, 68–71, 75,
77. *See also* Frequency shift
information

Doppler shift frequency—*continued*
  analysis of, 97–107
  bats' determination of, 12
  detection of, 95–97
  and flow velocity, 166
  lowering, as solution for aliasing, 130
  maximum, conversion to maximum blood
      velocity, 159
  methods of obtaining, 75
  and motion of echo source, 135
  and nonaxial flow, 72–73, 73f
  and velocity estimation, 174
Doppler signal analysis, 10, 78, 86–87
Doppler signal mix, 97
  source of, 78–82, 80f
Doppler signal processing
  limitations of, 143–152
  in M/Q system, 112
  steps in, 75–87
Doppler ultrasound. *See also* Pulsed Doppler
      ultrasound
  application goals, 13–15
  audio information, 133
  common problems of, 15
  diagnostic value of, 9
  effective penetration of, 27
  growth of, 9
  measurement errors, sources of, 71, 73f
  penetration, and frequency, 29
  signal separation problem in, 94–95, 96f
Doppler ultrasound technology
  applications of, 3–4
  correlation with invasive techniques, 177
Driving pressure, and volume flow, 139, 139f,
      156
Duplex imaging, 4
  of atherosclerotic cervical cerebrovascular
      disease, 7
  detection of extraluminal flow with, 6
  system
    advanced true, 118–127
    first true, 109–112
    organization, 109, 110f
  of vascular disease
    false positive rate for, 166
    sensitivity of, 166
    specificity of, 166

Echocardiography, 3–4, 7, 122–123
Echo signal, strength of, 15
Echo-signal phase, and direction, 92–95
Echo-signal processing, in nature, 11–12
Echo source
  accelerating, and Doppler shift frequency,
      135
  motion
    and Doppler shift frequency, 135

  echo signal phase with, in pulsed Dop-
      pler system, 85, 86f
  need to know, 13–14
Eddy currents, 44–45, 45f, 49, 55
  in blood flow, 58, 138, 138f, 139, 141
  with wall irregularities, 141
Embolic obstruction, Doppler sound patterns
      with, 3

f. See Frequency
Fast Fourier transform, 87, 101f, 101–107,
      112, 134, 155
  and complex numbers, 104–107
  digital display format, 102, 102f
Fat
  reflectivity in decibels below perfect reflec-
      tor, 23t
  ultrasound propagation velocity and at-
      tenuation rates for, 19t
Fat (eye), ultrasound propagation velocity and
      attenuation rates for, 19t
FFT. *See* Fast Fourier transform
Flow. *See also* Flow reversals
  character of, assumptions about, 173–174
  concepts of, 156–158
  direction of, 14–15
  nonaxial, 174
  spatial characterization of, 14
  temporal characteristics of, 14
Flow events, 134–143
Flow patterns. *See also* Jet(s)
  angiodynography of, 150, 157, 175
  assumptions about, 149–150
  in cardiac cycle, 135–137
  color flow imaging of, 150–151, 157, 163,
      165, 174–175
  effect of blood viscosity on, 165, 175–176
  multiphasic, 136
  and vessel stenosis, 174
Flow resistance, 14
Flow reversals, 14–15
  in blood flow, 58, 136–137, 138f
  regional, 15
Flow separations, 48, 50–51, 50f–51f
  in blood flow, 58, 140–141
  in carotid bulb, 50–51, 51f
  geometry of, 140, 140f
  poststenotic, 138, 138f
Flow velocity. *See* Fluid flow, velocity
Fluid behavior, and quantitation, 156
Fluid column, pressure from, 36–37, 37f
Fluid flow. *See also* Pulsatile flow
  with in-line turbulence, 49, 49f
  laminar. *See* Laminar flow
  Newtonian, 48
  parabolic, 48, 49f
  rate, in volume per unit time, 157

resistance to, 42–43, 55
   energy loss through, 53
spatial average velocity of, 157
stability of, 43–45, 47, 55
stable, in pipe, 48
unstable, 45f, 49–51, 55
velocity, 14, 41, 47–51, 55
   blunt profile, 49, 49f, 137
   and lumen narrowing, 45–46
   parabolic profile, 48, 49f, 137, 138f
Fluids
   distribution of applied pressure in, 38, 39f
   friction within, 47
   incompressibility, 37, 41
   inertia of, 54
   mass of, 36, 156
   in motion, 35, 40, 54–55. *See also* Fluid
      flow
      energy gradients of, 54–55
   moving through pipes, 41–55
   pressure in, as potential energy, 51–52
   pressure movement through, 39
   pressure propagation measurements in,
      39–40
   at rest, 35–40
   theory of, 35
   thickness, 35
   viscosity of, 43, 47–48
      measurement of, 47, 48f
Forward flow, 15
Fourier analysis, 97, 101. *See also* Fast
      Fourier transform
Fourier frequency components, 97, 101
   amplitude of. *See also* Gray scale
      proportionality to number of RBCs trav-
      eling together in same way, 102, 135
   mathematical estimation of, 155
   use of, in calculation of other parameters,
      155
Fourier pulsatility index, 170–171
Frequency
   of Doppler shift signal, 14
   and wavelength, 18
Frequency analysis
   complex number, 106f, 128
   real number, 106f, 128
Frequency bins, 102, 134
Frequency shift information, processing, 2

Grating lobes, 117, 118f
Gray scale, 102, 134–135, 176

Hand-held Doppler device, use and misuse
      of, 1–3
Heart
   flow in, 59–60, 130

as pump, evaluation of, 57, 155, 158–159
subcostal view, flow patterns in, 124f
Heart muscle, ultrasound propagation ve-
      locity and attenuation rates for, 19t
Heart valve(s)
   area of, estimation of, 163–165
   evaluation of, 158–159
   flow through, 161
   function, 143
   pressure gradients across, 161–163
   regurgitation, evaluation of, 159
   stenotic, 4
      flow through, 161–162
      pressure gradient across, measurement
         of, 159
Hematocrit
   regional changes in, and reflectivity of
      blood, 25
   and ultrasound scattering, 23, 24f
Hematomas, periarterial, 6
Hemodynamics, 35. *See also* Blood flow
Heterodyning, 93, 94f
Hue, 120
Hydraulic gain, in fluid, 38–39, 39f
Hydraulic reflections, 136–137
Hydrodynamics, 35, 40
   summary of, 54–55
Hydrostatic pressure, 52
   independence of direction, 37
Hydrostatic pressure equation, 36–37
Hydrostatics, 35–40
   first fluid paradox of, 36f, 36–37
   first law of, 37
   second fluid paradox of, 38, 38f
Hypertension, 46

I channel, 85, 93
Imaginary numbers, 104
Imaging goals, 13, 13t
Innominate artery, mistaken for ascending
      aorta, 176–177
In-phase channel. *See* I channel
Internal carotid artery, stenosis, estimation
      of, 167

Jet(s)
   deviations of, 149–150
   direction of, in velocity estimation,
      174–175
   effect of blood viscosity on, 165
   formation of, assumptions about, 162–163
   geometry of, 149, 150f, 162–163, 174
   non-axial, geometry of, 149, 150f
   position of, determination of, 174
   from stenosis, 159
      assumptions about, 149
   velocity of, measurement of, 162–163

Keagy algorithm, 167–169, 168f
Kidney
    reflectivity in decibels below perfect reflector, 23t
    ultrasound propagation velocity and attenuation rates for, 19t
Kinetic energy, in fluids, 51–52

Lagging signals, 93
λ. *See* Wavelength
Laminar flow, 48, 49f, 55
    of blood, 137, 138f
Laplace transforms, 173
Leading signals, 93
Left ventricular filling
    flow through mitral valve in, 142, 144f
    vortex formation in, 141–142, 142f
Left ventricular outflow tract, flow through, 142, 145f
Lens effect, caused by shaped interfaces, 30, 30f
Limb ischemia, Doppler sound patterns with, 3
Linear transducer arrays. *See also* Phased array transducers, linear
    focusing, 151
Liver
    diseased, ultrasound propagation velocity and attenuation rates for, 19t
    normal, ultrasound propagation velocity and attenuation rates for, 19t
    reflectivity in decibels below perfect reflector, 23t
Liver-blood interface, reflection from, 27f
Liver-fat interface, reflection from, 27f
Logarithmic amplifier, compression in, 79f
Low-pass filtering, 104
Lung, ultrasound propagation velocity and attenuation rates for, 19t

Master oscillator circuit, 82–83
Master oscillator signal, in-phase and out-of-phase, 93
Mean pulsatility index, 170, 172
Mitral valve
    area, estimation of, 163–165, 165f
    leaflets
        multiple motion of, 142, 143f
        passive closure of, with ventricular filling, 142, 143f
    M-mode imaging of, 142
    pressure gradient across, 162
    real-time imaging of, 142
    in ventricular filling, 142, 144f
M-mode display, 110
M-mode imaging
    of aortic diameter, 176
    of mitral valve, 142

MO circuit. *See* Master oscillator circuit
M/Q organization, 110–112
M/Q system, 109–112
    organization of, 112f
Multifilter analysis, 87, 98f, 98–99
Multiphasic flow patterns, 136
Muscle, reflectivity in decibels below perfect reflector, 23t
MVA. See Mitral valve, area
Myocardial infarction, and diagnostic value of Doppler devices, 3

Neural tissue, ultrasound propagation velocity and attenuation rates for, 19t
Newton, Isaac, 48
Newtonian fluids, 48
Nonstructural echoes, 15–16
Nyquist frequency, 71
Nyquist limit, 103, 126–127
    removal of, in Doppler signal processing, 128

Obstructive disease. *See also* Atherosclerotic plaque; Vessel stenosis
    spectral broadening with, 147, 149f
Operating frequency, lowering, as solution for aliasing, 130

P. See Hydrostatic pressure
Panamanian mustache bat, use of Doppler effect, 11–12
Parabolic velocity profile, 48, 49f, 156
    of blood, 137, 138f
Pascal's law, 38, 39f, 54
Peak-to-peak pulsatility index, 170–171, 171f
Penetration
    and reflection and attenuation, 25–29
    and system gain, 27
    and system output, 27
Periarterial abscess, 6
Peripheral arteries, occlusion, Doppler sound patterns with, 3
Peripheral vascular disease, evaluation of, 173
Phantoms, testing with, 144–145
Phase angle, 96–97
Phased array transducers
    in duplex imaging, 117
    focusing, 151, 152f
    linear, 90, 91f, 122
        beam focusing, 117, 117f, 151, 152f
        beam steering, 117, 117f
        in duplex system, 117
Phaser diagram, 76–77, 78f, 94–95, 96f
Phase-sensitive detection, 23, 24f
Phase shift
    negative, 92–93
    positive, 92–93

Platelets, physical characteristics of, 56–57
Poise, 43
Poiseuille's equation, 42, 55
Pourcelot's ratio, 14, 170–172, 172f
Pressure, in fluids, as potential energy, 51–52
Pressure-flow relationship, 42f, 43–44
PRF. *See* Pulse repetition frequency
Propagating medium, 17
Propagation velocity, 17–18, 64
    of ultrasound, 64
    for various tissues, 18, 19t
Pseudoaneurysm
    characteristic hydrodynamic pattern of, 6
    with transarterial catheterization, 6
Pulmonary artery, blunt velocity profile in,
        141
Pulsatile flow, 54–55, 55f
    in vascular system, 57
Pulsatile function, average value of, calcula-
        tion of, 158f
Pulsatility, measurement of, for vascular eval-
        uations, 170
Pulsatility index, 14, 170. *See also* Fourier
        pulsatility index; Mean pulsatility in-
        dex; Peak-to-peak pulsatility index
Pulsed Doppler duplex system, 114–118
    common transducer, 115–116, 116f
    outboard, 115, 115f
Pulsed Doppler system, 75. *See also* Quadra-
        ture phase detection
    coherent, 82, 84f
    controlled transmission in, 82–84
    Doppler detector, 86
    Doppler signal analysis, 86–87
    echo signal phase with echo source motion,
        85, 86f
    effective aliasing limit, 107
    forward and reverse channels, 85–86, 93.
        See also I channel; Q channel
    frequency divider, 83
    frequency limits, 103
    gated transmitter circuit, 83
    master oscillator circuit. *See* Master os-
        cillator circuit
    range gate in, 91f, 91–92
    range of Doppler shift frequencies, 81
    receiver, 84–85
    sampling fields for, 83f
    signal separation problem in, 95
    spatial resolution with, 82–87
Pulsed Doppler ultrasound, 14
    burst length, 11–12
    determination of real velocity profile by,
        156–157
    sampling limit of, 71
Pulsed wave Doppler system. *See* Pulsed
        Doppler system
Pulse repetition frequency, 32–33, 83, 125
    in estimation of Doppler shift frequency, 96

increasing, as solution for aliasing,
        128–129
    and MO frequency, relationship between,
        83, 85f
    and Nyquist limit, 103

Q. See Volume flow
Q channel, 86, 93
QPD. *See* Quadrature phase detector
Q transducer, 76
Quadrature channel. *See* Q channel
Quadrature phase detection, 77, 85–86, 93,
        94f, 95
Quadrature phase detector, 111–112
Quality-factor, 76
Quantitation
    in cardiology, 158–173
    errors, 173–177
    and fluid behavior, 156
    logical and calculation traps in, 173–177
    overview of, 155–156

R. See Reflection coefficient
Range ambiguity artifact, 32f, 32–33, 92,
        92f
Range-gate position, measurement of,
        144–145
Range gating, 82
    techniques, 90–92
RBCs. *See* Red blood cell(s)
Real-time systems, frame rates in, 32–33
Red blood cell(s)
    aggregates of, as source of blood echo sig-
        nals, 24f, 24–25
    diameter of, 24
    in motion, and Fourier component ampli-
        tude, 102, 135
    organization of flow, and range of Doppler
        shift frequencies, 81–82
    physical characteristics of, 56
    in ultrasound applications of Doppler,
        69–70
    ultrasound scattering from, 56
Reflection(s). *See also* Hydraulic reflections
    at interfaces, 18–22
    and penetration, 25–29
Reflection coefficient, 19
Reflector attenuation line
    biological, 25–26, 27f
    maximum, 25, 26f
Refraction, 20f, 29f, 29–30
Region of maximum sensitivity, 76
    formation of, 89–90, 90f
Resistance, to flow. *See* Fluid flow,
        resistance to
Reverberations, 30–31, 31f
Reversed flow. *See* Flow reversals

Reynolds, Osborne, 43–44
Reynolds equation, 44
Reynolds number, 44, 55
Roederer-Strandness algorithm, 168–169, 169f
Rouleaux, 56
R-R interval, 159
    average flow over, 159, 160f

Sample volume
    accuracy of, 144–146
    at edge of flow velocity gradient, 147, 148f
    geometry of, 151–152
    with in-line turbulence, 147, 148f–149f
    lateral size of, 151
    size, 156–157
    small, with high velocity, 147, 148f
    in turning streamline, 147, 148f
Sampling, 104
    digital, harmonic frequency generation with, 104, 105f
    and high-frequency aliasing, 125
    for synchronous color flow imaging, 119f
Scatter, in Doppler data, 174
Scattering, 19–21, 20f
    from blood, 23
    as function of hematocrit, 23, 24f
    off surface irregularities, 21–22
    signal amplitude reduction in, 21f
    ultrasonic energy lost in, 22
Scattering bodies, 18
Scattering site size, 25
Scattering units, dimensions of, 22
Sector scanning field, in color flow imaging, 122, 123f
Separation bubbles, 140
Shadowing, 31–32
Shear forces, 47f, 47–48
Sideband-filtering techniques, 95
Signal compression, 27–29
Signal processing, 15
    asynchronous, 110, 118–120
    in continuous wave Doppler system, 76–78
    details of, 89–107
    parallel, 118, 122
    steps in, 75–87
    synchronous, 109, 118–119
Signal separation problem, in Doppler ultrasound, 94–95, 96f
Skeletal muscle
    lens effect of, 30
    ultrasound propagation velocity and attenuation rates for, 19t
Skull, ultrasound propagation velocity and attenuation rates for, 19t
Snell's law, 30
Soft tissue, reflectivity in decibels below perfect reflector, 23t

Sonograph, design of, 13
Spatial average, of velocity profile, calculation of, 157–158, 159f
Speckling effect, 23, 24f
Spectral broadening
    sources of, 140–141, 146–147, 166
    in normal blood flow, 148f–149f
    with vessel stenosis, 147, 148f–149f
Spectral content, and flow angle, 150–151
Spectral display(s), 133
    basic components of, 134f
    elements of, 134–135
    improvement of, 176
    and motion elements, 135
Spectral output, real view of, 146–147
Specular reflection, 19–20, 20f
    amplitude, with changing angle of incidence, 20, 21f
Spleen, ultrasound propagation velocity and attenuation rates for, 19t
Stenosis. *See* Vessel stenosis
Streamlines, 44, 55
    breakup of, 147
    energy along, 51–52
    in stable flow, 51
    with unstable flow, 50
String phantom, testing with, 144–145, 146f
Stroke distance, 160–161
Stroke volume
    and cardiac output, 160
    determination of, 159–161
    measurement of, problems in, 176
Superficial femoral artery, flow events in, 135f
Surface irregularities, scattering off, 21–22
SV. See Stroke volume
System gain, 27
System leakage signal, 76–77
System power control, 27

TGC. *See* Time-gain compensation
Thermal dilution, correlation with Doppler ultrasound, 177
Θ. *See* Cosine Θ; Doppler angle
Thrombocytes, physical characteristics of, 56–57
Time-average flow velocity, calculation of, 159, 160f
Time-gain compensation, 27–29
Time-share duplex imaging, 110, 111f, 112–118
Tissue attenuation, 15, 29. *See also* Attenuation rates, for various tissues, 19t
Tissue reflectivity dynamic range, 22–23
Tissue-ultrasound interaction, 17–33
Transducers, 89–90. *See also* Annular transducer array; Phased array transducers

for continuous wave Doppler systems, 75–76
focusing, 151, 152f
in true duplex system, 110
undamped, 76
Transducer-skin interface, coupling between, 32
Tricuspid valve, pressure gradient across, 162
Turbulence
in blood flow, 139
poststenotic, 138f, 138–139

Ultrasound
applications of, 7
common problems in, 15–16
imaging goals, 13, 13t
interpretation of, 7
as mechanical wave, 17–18
and tissue, interactions between, 33

Valvular stenosis. *See* Heart valve(s), stenotic
Vascular compartment, flow in, assumptions about, 149–150
Vascular disease
estimation of, 166–173
spectral output with, 146–147
Vascular system
flexible, model of blood flow in, 57
geometry of flow within, 72, 73f
hydraulic response of, 57
physical characteristics of, 57
Vc. See Critical velocity equation
Vector component, 66
Velocity, computation of, 174–176
Velocity profile. *See also* Blunt velocity profile; Parabolic velocity profile
across vessel lumen, 156
spatial average of, calculation of, 157–158, 159f
Venous pressure, 37–38
Ventricular emptying. *See also* Ventricular outflow
flow events in, 142–143
Ventricular filling, 59
flow events in, 141–142
vortex formation in, 59, 141–142, 142f
Ventricular outflow, 59–60
flow events in, 142–143
Venturi effect, 52, 57, 140
Vessel diameter
and flow resistance, 43

and volume, 43
Vessel narrowing
and blood flow, 138–139
gradual, smooth, 140
Vessel stenosis
assumptions about flow in, 149–150
blood flow at, 58, 59f, 138f, 138–139
flow disturbances produced by, 166
and flow patterns, 174
geometry of, 149
spectral broadening with, 147, 148f–149f
velocity profiles at, 138f
Viscosity, 43
Viscous forces, 43
Volume flow, 14, 41–55
determination of, 157–158
and driving pressure, 139, 139f
effect of velocity on, 47
as function of applied pressure, 42, 42f
model of, expansion of, 45–46
through rigid pipe, 41f
Volumetric flow, 2–3
Vortices, 44–45, 45f, 49, 55
in blood flow, 58, 138f, 139, 141
in ventricular filling, 59, 141–142, 142f

Wall irregularities, effect on blood flow, 140–141
Water. *See also* Fluids
reflectivity in decibels below perfect reflector, 23t
Wavelength
calculation of, 18
and frequency, 18
Wavelength-frequency equation, 64, 69
Wave propagation, 64
and constant wave velocity, 64, 64f
isotropic, 64, 64f
symmetrical, 64, 64f
Wave properties, 17
WBCs. *See* White blood cells
White blood cells, physical characteristics of, 56
Windkessel model, 57

Z. See Acoustic impedance
ZCD. *See* Zero-crossing detector
Zero-crossing detector, 87, 99–101, 134
error production in, 100, 100f
frequency approximation with, 99, 99f
Zero-shift, 126–127